GOD-GIVEN HERBS

FOR THE HEALING

OF MANKIND

Consultant in Herbal and Nutritional Therapy

(C) Library of Congress No. Ai-11916

ISB NO. 0-9617405-9

Copies available from your local bookstore
or by mailorder.

S. Chupp's Books

G-27539 Londick

Burr Oak, Michigan 49030

FOREWORD BY THE AUTHOR, 15 YEARS LATER:

When I first wrote this book, in 1970, there was just beginning to I a wider interest in the use of herbs. This interest coincided with tI increasing awareness by the public that orthodox medicine wa neither the only nor even likely always the *best* answer to illness.

Since ancient times, when Hippocrates, the Father of Medicir first stated "If you can cure the patient with foods and exercise, lea your drugs in the chemist's pot," there has been a popular antipathy expensive drugs.

The tendency of any professional class is to make its profession mysterious realm with NO ADMITTANCE signs out for amateurs. Bi it is true that your body does not belong to the doctor, it is yc responsibility to decide what you want done to your body. E lightened laymen have a constitutional right to treat themselves they wish. Claiming his rights to his own body, a friend of mine w entered a hospital recently, suffering from abdominal pain, demand to be released when doctors told him they would use explorat surgery. Even though they protested, he signed himself out of t hospital and soon recovered by using a simple home remedy.

The ancient Hippocratic school of medicine in Greece trained physicians (like Luke, the beloved doctor) to believe that in any c *nature* (that is, the powers and constitution of the body, under Go blessing) is the principal healer. All that the physician can do remove or reduce the impediments to this natural defense a recuperation. Hence Hippocratic treatment made little use of dru but depended chiefly upon fresh air, emetics, suppositories, enem: poultices, ointments, massage, sweat and steam baths. Hippocra prescribed prayer as an aid but placed much reliance on sim therapies.

Use of pragmatic natural therapies should not be confused w pagan pantheism, in which nature itself is worshipped. One of unfortunate things about the modern holistic movement is that i often confused with uncritical acceptance of any therapy, includ occult, Hindu, powpowing, sorcery, and even superstitious practi:

i

such as the use of divining devices (pendulum, etc.). It is clear that the Christian will avoid such questionable practises like the plague.

However, another extreme would be that of "witch-hunting" bigots who try to smear all natural therapies as pantheistic or superstitious. A somewhat extreme book on this subject has been written by J. Weldon and C. Wilson, entitled "Occult Shock and Psychic Forces," 1980. Even this book admits there is room for a *distinctively Christian holistic health.* They state that providing the eastern-occult methods and philosophies are rejected, *what remains is sound.*

The sound core of the holistic health movement is the emphasis on preventive medicine, less reliance on drugs and surgery, advocating more personal responsibility for one's health, treating the cause instead of the symptom, etc.

We challenge all Christian readers to put any health therapy to a simple test, is it something conformable to Bible revelation or contrary to it? Is it something natural and pragmatic, like diet, herbs, massage, etc., or is it occult and weird? Through ignorance or bigotry, there are some who dismiss anything that seems strange to them. For example, some dismiss homeopathy as "occult" because they cannot believe that so small an amount of plant substance could act as a remedy. But it is a scientific fact that one plant extract made only with water was discovered which had a remarkable effect on the agglutination of red blood cells, with only *one* part of the plant fluid to 16,000 parts of water! Clearly, this is not a case of demons in the plants but practical chemistry.

Similarly, some have dismissed all acupuncture as "occult" because of its oriental origin. Yet acupuncture is even now widely used by veterinarians for the treatment of horses! Are we to assume that the horses will be affected by oriental philosophies and religions?

One area in which the Plain People need to exercise much more caution, is in the inherited superstitious practises of "pow-powing." It is our belief that any "spells," use of black threads and burning fires, are elements of black magic and should not be meddled with by born-again Christians. "Witching," divining, and such-like hocus pocus should be discarded. If it is not bordering on the occult it is on the superstitious. I met a man, for example, who was trying to locate a good real estate property by dangling a pendulum over a map! Such credibility argues that a person had abdicated common sense!

Another area of lunatic fringe interests in the health field can be seen in the "pyramid" craze, where people have gone around promoting the use of "pyramid" structures to "concentrate cosmic energy." There are many charlatans in the health field. Many schemes are obviously money-making schemes and will help the health of nobody but the promoter's pocket book!

Christians should remember to visit the sick, pray for the healing of the sick, and not neglect God-given herbs *or* good doctors!

The most important thing to consider, in visiting any health practitioner, is that you prove all things by the Word of God. Can you entrust your health and that of your family to men who are atheistic, occult or pantheistic? We have heard of numerous cases of spiritual damage which overcame and confused or even destroyed those who consulted palm readers, hypnotists, agnostic psychologists and psychiatrists, or witch doctors.

Even well-meaning practitioners can be betrayed into foolish practises by their indiscriminating professionalism. Hundreds of medical doctors prescribed thalidomide for pregnant women in Europe, because they trusted the chemical manufacturers of the drug who had claimed to have tested it and found it "harmless." But the manufacturer had lied in order to make more profit. The result was thousands of babies born with seal-like flippers instead of normal arms and legs.

Many are now questioning the practise of dentists using mercury-laden fillings for tooth cavities. Medical doctors continue to use many varieties of high-powered drugs with known bad side-effects. Each year hundreds die from tranquillizer abuse yet tranquillizers remain one of the most widely prescribed durgs. Whose fault is it?

Each year, a million and a half babies are aborted before birth. Does not the very ground cry out when it is stained with innocent blood? Who is prescribing and carrying out abortions? Who is prescribing birth control pills to make sex easy for unmarrieds? Is this not a species of quackery, too? Is this not a pagan sacrifice on the altar of Moloch or some other modern idol? Let the medical profession beware lest it shed innocent blood like pagans of old!

DID YOU KNOW?

Did you know that mankind would perish without herbs and plants? All of our food comes either directly from plants and their products or from animals which feed upon plants. The U.S. Department of Agriculture estimates that 60 to 67 percent of the average American diet comes directly from plant crops and the livestock products which make up the remaining 33 to 40 percent come from plants indirectly. The Bible clearly states in the first chapter of the first book that man is dependent on plants and herbs for food and meat (see page 3).

Did you know that without green plants purifying the air of the earth, few living things could even exist on the earth's surface? Plants absorb carbon dioxide and liberate oxygen and help maintain earth's atmosphere by photosynthesis and respiration, so that man can breathe the breath of life. Man is dependent on God-given plants to purify the air.

Did you know that plants take the radiant energy of the light of the sun and transform it into organic energy which man can then eat and absorb? The more light radiation contained in your food the more life energy you will have — man is dependent on live foods for vitamins essential to health (see page 78).

Did you know that plants of the past, buried, altered, preserved and yielding coal, oil and natural gas, as well as plants of the present provide the Key materials for light, heat and fuel? Again we see how God has made man dependent on plants.

Did you know that furthermore God prescribed plants to be used as medicines for mankind? (See page 3). Did you know that plant medicines are frequently superior to and safer than synthetic medicines (see pages 21, 38, 40)?

Did you know that God created man to live in a beautiful garden of plants and that man is never really content divorced from the beauty and refreshment of the plants of field and forest?

Did you know that despite all of man's scientific advance there is little possibility that he can free himself from this dependence on plants? All the energy required to keep us alive and most of the energy required to run our industries comes directly or indirectly from God-given plants, trees and herbs.

GOD-GIVEN HERBS FOR THE HEALING OF MANKIND

by William R. McGrath

"And God said, Behold, I have given you every herb bearing seed, which is upon the face of all the earth; and every tree; in which is the fruit of a tree yielding seed; to you it shall be for meat".
—(Genesis 1:29).

". . . And the fruit thereof shall be for meat, and the leaf thereof for medicine."—(Ezekiel 47:12).

"He causeth the grass to grow for the cattle, and herb(s) for the service of man; that He may bring forth food out of the earth."
—(Psalm 104:14).

"And Isaiah said, Take a (poultice) of figs. And they took and laid it on the boil, and (King Hezekiah) recovered."—(II. Kings 20:7).

"The Lord hath created medicines out of the earth; and he that is wise will not abhor them."—(Apocryphal Book of Ecclesiasticus 38:4).

"For one believeth he may eat all things; another who is weak eateth herbs."—(Romans 14:2).

"And he shewed me a pure river of water of life, clear as crystal, proceeding out of the throne of God and of the Lamb. In the midst of the street of it, and on either side of the river, was there the tree of life, which bare twelve manner of fruits, and yielded her fruit every month: and the leaves of the tree were for the healing of the nations". (Revelation 22:1,2).

Herbs have been used for medicine since time immemorial. The Bible itself records God's prescription of herbs for the healing of mankind. This present book was written to briefly tell the history of the use of herbs for medicinal purposes. Hippocrates, the ancient Greek Father of Medicine said: "Your food shall be your medicine, and your medicine shall be your food." This is why one should take herbs for prevention, for building up body defenses and for the maintenance of health, and not only for cures. The closer our foods are to that which is natural, the more opportunity our bodies will have to work as they were designed. Nature was the first drugstore. There are many artificial foods and many strong, synthetic chemical drugs, but there is no satisfactory substitute for herbs. God has prescribed, and surely His prescription is perfect.

TABLE OF CONTENTS

Ginseng 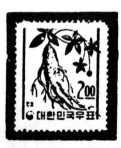 Plant

First Printing: February, 1970
Second Printing: April, 1970
Third Printing: September, 1970
Fourth Printing: January, 1971
Fifth Printing: March 1972
Sixth Printing: 1981
Seventh Printing: 1986
Eight Printing: 1988
Ninth Printing: April 1998
Printed in U.S.A.

This book was written because of the author's personal experience of being healed from an arthritic condition by the help of herbs and it is now launched in the fond hope that it will be helpful to those curious about various old-fashioned natural cures obtained from herbs and plants. This information is not presented with the intention of diagnosing or prescribing, but only offered to help you cooperate with your doctor in your mutual desire to build and maintain your health. In the event you use this information without your doctor's approval, you are prescribing for yourself, which is your constitutional right, but no responsibility is assumed on the part of the author, publisher or distributors of the book. It is not the purpose of this book to replace the service of your physician. By all means see a doctor for any condition which requires his services. Nor does this book promote the sale of any patent medicines, endorse the sale or consumption of any medicinal or nutritional preparations nor guarantee the effectiveness of any recipe. The purpose of this book is to edify and enlighten the general reader, not to sell medicines or advance any claim for medical omniscience or infallibility. The various herb recipes mentioned in this book are culled from herb books, ancient and modern, and the reporting herein of how they have been historically used as remedies and treatments does not constitute any unqualified endorsement or guarantee of cure. We doubt if the use of simple home remedies could or should ever be eliminated. Nor should home remedies ever make doctors and physicians obsolete. Herbs, like all good, natural foods, are preventive remedies full of vitamins, minerals, hormones and enzymes. If we made more use of them, we would need to impose less on the time of our busy doctors. The well-known American naturalist, Henry David Thoreau, wrote: "A man may esteem himself happy when that which is his food is also his medicine." In a day when the asphalt jungles of the modern city are spreading like a blight over our polluted planet, and it is popular to indiscriminately exterminate wild plants by herbicides, many city dwellers irrationally fear and despise all wild flora as "weeds". But herbs have been used since the beginning of recorded time for medicinal and nutritional purposes and modern scientific research has proven that plants contain many remarkable healing properties. That is the subject of this book. For those who wish to study the subject more in detail, numerous books for further reference are cited in this book. We invite readers to correspond with us if they have any additional interesting herbal home remedies, or if they note any errors in this book needing correction.

CHAPTER I: What the Bible Says About Sickness and Health:

Talk with anyone about sickness and health and you will soon discover people have strong likes and dislikes, prejudices and convictions, from numerous personal experiences. We have all been sick; we all want to be healthy. We all seem to have pet peeves and favorite remedies. We all know of friends or acquaintances who became health faddists or fanatics, specializing in one narrow extreme to the exclusion of all other approaches.

We realize people can get so narrow-minded on the subject of health and sickness that they blindly close their eyes to any type of treatment apart from one pet type. If people were always reasonable, they would be open to considering the value of various types of medical treatments and accept whatever was most helpful. I have written this book primarily out of my own experience of having been healed of a crippling arthritic condition which conventional medical treatment was unable to help. My health problem responded marvelously to treatment by an age-old method known since Bible times and practised down through the ages among simple people living close to nature. It is a shame that the ancient methods of herbal therapy have been so neglected in our times. Fortunately there is a great revival of interest now in such methods.

MANKIND IS IN TROUBLE

Is it not often the case that mankind seems to get into such terrible difficulties through depending on the feeble light of human reasoning and then turns back in desperation to the Bible for help? Modern man in his pride and presumption has brought the world to the very edge of atomic destruction, to the threshold of planet-wide air and water pollution, to militarism and dictatorship. Now man sits up and takes notice of the terrible situation he has brought upon himself and wonders where to turn to next. Long ago the BIBLE predicted such a situation would come in the end times. Just as the world is in such a mess politically and socially today through want of trying the Bible prescription for peace and joy available in Christ, so we also believe the deplorable state of health among men, with the spreading plagues of cancer, heart disease, rheumatism, etc., could be greatly relieved by a return to Biblical prescriptions in the area of healthful living.

We would not want to be misunderstood to be saying or claiming that modern medical science should be abandoned in favor of a return to merely ancient medicine. Rather what we mean is that the divine wisdom of the Bible, predating modern medicine by many thousands of years, still has a relevant remedy for the sickness of mankind. Medical science recognizes that such emotions as fear, sorrow, envy, resentment and hatred are responsible for the majority of our sicknesses. Emotional stress can cause such serious diseases as migraine headache, apoplexy, heart trouble, ulcers, high blood pressure, insanity, etc. Physicians prescribe medicines for the symptoms of these diseases but cannot cure the underlying cause: emotional stress and strain and confusion. It is in precisely such "medically modern" countries as the United States that we find a tremendous increase in psychosomatic diseases brought on by a fast, artificial, stress-laden and anxiety-ridden rat-race, giving Americans the world's highest incidence of heart trouble, cancer, insanity and other degenerative diseases of body and soul. Artificial foods, poisonous saturation of the countryside with super-powerful insecticides, increasing air pollution, improvident wasting of the natural resources, nervous tension, multiplied immorality, the changeover to a permanent war-time state, the growing cult of violence, —all these are taking their toll.

But what is most disquieting is not only that our modern medical science is failing to address itself effectively to the psychosomatic sicknesses of our time but it is often inept in trying to cope with the merely physical symptoms. Not only are our hospitals overcrowded and understaffed, medical insurance programs inadequate, prescription drugs overcharged, too many people financially ruined by medical bills, but there is a widespread feeling among the people that the level of professional services available is uneven and careless. Numerous exposures of graft, corruption, profiteering, ignorance, venality, unnecessary operations performed, and general incompetence of many medical doctors, are now being published, Such books as the following are only a few of the well-documented exposures revealing the glaring deficiencies of orthodox medicine: "THE AMERICAN HEALTH SCANDAL" (by Roul Tunley, Dell Publishing Co., 256 pp., 1966), "THE DOCTORS" (By Martin L. Gross, Dell Publishing Co., 718 pp., 1966), and "THE HEALERS (by Anonymous M.D., G. P. Putnam Publishers, 251 pp., 1967).

THE RETURN TO HERBAL MEDICINE

We mention these things not to run down the medical doctor or overlook the many unsung heroes among doctors who practice medicine as a sacrificial service to others instead of a profiteering self-service, but simply to remind our readers that medicine is a field which cannot afford a monopolistic approach by one clique of practitioners who claim to know it all and try to boycott or blackball all other approaches to medicine and healing. When herbal medicines are mentioned, for example, the average medical doctor tends to react emotionally and denounce all such things as on a level with witch doctors! But the simple fact is that the doctor himself is unwittingly using herbal medicines all the time — in 1963, out of more than 300 million prescriptions written by American doctors, more than 47% contained a medicine of natural origin as the principal ingredient, or one of the two main ingredients! Furthermore, the sale of medicines solely from botanical sources has increased five-fold in the period from 1950 to 1960 alone. In their desperation to find more effective cures, drug research companies are investing more and more millions of dollars in the search for medicinal plants and their derivatives. To those who are familiar with the Bible, this direction should come as no surprise —what is more surprising is that modern medical science has not gone back to herbal medicine earlier.

BACK TO THE BIBLE

In a well-known passage that antedated modern medical science by many thousands of years on the vital importance of herbs, the Bible says: "And God said, Behold, I have given you every herb bearing seed, which is upon the face of all the earth; and every tree; in which is the fruit of a tree yielding seed; to you it shall be for meat." (Genesis 1:29). Related Scriptures remind us: "and the fruit thereof shall be for meat, and the leaf thereof for medicine." (Ezekiel 47:12). "He causeth the grass to grow for the cattle, and herbs for the service of men; that he may bring forth food out of the earth." (Psalm 104:14). The apocryphal book of Ecclesiasticus (38:4) notes also: "The Lord hath created medicines out of the earth; and he that is wise will not abhor them." Those who believe the Bible to be God's Word believe that it is not merely accidental or insignificant to find such directions indicated for the source of more effective medicines. The Bible is after all the best Health Book on earth — it is primarily concerned with mankind's spiritual health, that men should turn from sin-sickness to find God's forgiveness and peace in Christ. This alone can cure the spiritual cancers of lust, greed, envy, hatred, resentment and warfare. But the Bible also contains secondary directions for the cure of the physical man by measures of simple, natural methods and medicines.

BACK TO NATURE

We would do well to remember that God is the God ruling over Nature. The 'father of Medical science', the Greek Hippocrates, maintained that all diseases are caused by the obstruction and perversion of Nature and can only be cured by Nature (with the doctor assisting!). Oliver Wendell Holmes went some further when he said, "Nature cures but the doctor collects the fee!" Understanding the natural basis of cure, we feel that natural therapies are superior and natural herbal medicines more easily assimilable by the body than synthetic medicines. We are living in a day when it is becoming more recognized that organic fertilizers (natural fertilizers) are better for your garden than highly synthetic chemical fertilizers that often have undesirable side-effects. Similarly, organic herbal medicines are easier on your body than synthetic chemical drugs with harsh side-effects.

Dr. Otto Mauset, in his book "HERBS FOR HEALTH", has well said: "Chemistry of today has accomplished wonderful results in many ways, but all the laboratories in the world will never be able to supplant the remarkable fine process which takes place in the living cell. They will never successfully imitate the wonderful methods that Nature uses in performing its work in the plant, as well as in the human body... Remedies from chemicals and minerals will never stand in favorable comparison with the products of Nature — the living cell of the plant, the final result of the ray of the sun, the mother of all life... When correctly used, herbs promote the elimination of waste matter and poisons from the system by simple natural means. They support Nature in its fight against disease; while chemicals, not being assimilable, add to the accumulation of morbid matter and only simulate improvement by suppressing the symptoms."

To recognize and appreciate the ancient medical wisdom of the Bible is not the same as gullibly endorsing ALL ancient or primitive medicine — much of which was simply atrocious superstition in the idolatrous religions of the ancient world. Take for example the ancient Egyptian medical treatise called the PAPYRUS EBERS — it prescribed such fantastic and debased concoctions as magic water poured over idols, the dung of dogs, cats and flies, etc. But Moses, who was well-versed in all the wisdom of the Egyptians, was directed by God to write down a system of superbly simple and natural medicine which was based on sanitation, quarantine of infectious cases, cleanliness, avoidance of dangerous and contaminated foods, strict scrubbing after contact with dead or diseased persons, etc. It was a sanitary system 3,500 years ahead of modern medical science and possible only by divine inspiration! As late as 1876, tens of thousands were still dying yearly and unnecessarily in European and American hospitals for lack of a simple system of sanitation and cleanliness. Doctors would turn unwashed from an autopsy on a dead person to directly delivering a baby and then wonder why both mother and child frequently died!

BIBLE SANITATION AND SANITY

The Old Testament contains numerous and detailed prescriptions legislating the requirements for clean hands and feet, clean bodies, clean clothing, clean personal habits, clean foods, clean homes, clean morals, clean spirits, clean worship and clean customs. Cleanliness and purity of body and spirit were then (and still are) the essentials of holiness. All of it together is well summarised in the New Testament teaching: "Know ye not that your body is the temple of the Holy Ghost which is in you, ... and ye are not your own? For ye are bought with a price; therefore glorify God in your body, and in your spirit, which are God's. If any man defile the temple of God, him shall God destroy; for the temple of God is holy, which temple ye are... Whether therefore ye eat, or drink, or whatsoever ye do, do all to the glory of God." (I. Corinthians 6:19-20, 3:17, 10:31). These simple yet comprehensive commandments on purity of heart, mind and body would mandatorily eliminate those common modern health menances of alcoholism, venereal disease, tobacco indulgence, drug addiction, and coronary collapse from over-indulgence in gluttony. (The Old Testament specifically forbade the eating of blood or fat —two substances very susceptible of transmitting disease and overloading the cardio-vascular system). Also the Bible command to set apart one day out of seven, as a day of rest, ensured a wonderful weekly vacation from the killing pace, the stress and strain of materialism. Cleanliness, purity, moderation, simplicity and rest added up to a simple prescription for sanity and health.

THE BIBLE AS A HEALTH BOOK

The Bible as a Health Book is pre-eminently modern in its medical approach, botanically, naturally and spiritually. The Bible recognizes disease as an inevitable accompaniment of human life but gives copious directions on how to live the happy and peaceful life free of unnecessary psychosomatic diseases. The Bible teaches simple, pure, natural living as the way of spiritual and physical health but it also teaches the recourse of divine intervention by supernatural healing in exceptional cases. Christ during His earthly ministry was much occupied in the ministry of healing, as were also the apostles and the early Christians. Showing again and again the often intimate connection between physical illness and psychosomatic causes, Christ and the Early Church emphasized confession of sins, forgiveness, and then physical healing. However there was no fanatical teaching that right living would ennable one to evade dying physically. Instead, salvation was experienced through forgiveness of sins and spiritual regeneration ("being born again") and eventual death was anticipated as a release from mortality to the greater liberty of immortality. The Christian picture of Heaven includes an ultimate renovation of the earth itself, banishment of death, restoration of a Garden of Eden and redeemed mankind living forever around the Tree of Life, whose leaves were for the healing of the nations (Revelation 22:1,2). Whether this is meant symbolically or not, the Bible picture of immortality includes a portrayal of the Tree of Life with its healing leaves! Note the tie between leaves and healing.

The Bible is a realistic Book on the subject of health and sickness, as well as on all other topics too. It does not promise sinful mankind any kind of magic pill to save them IN their sins but offers a Saviour Who saves men FROM their sins and directs them in a simple, pure way of life lived in harmony with God's plan of nature. This plan includes doctors (Luke was after all called the "beloved physician"), herbal medicines, foods, rest, sane living, purity, prayer and basic dependence upon the Great Physician, Christ. All of these methods of healing were in use by the people of the Bible. Yet the Bible also mentions the danger of medical incompetence: "A certain woman, ... had suffered many things of many physicians, and had spent all that she had, and was nothing bettered, but rather grew worse." (Mark 5:26). In her desperation she turned from these to a strong faith that only Christ could heal her, and healed she was. It is this writer's belief that the sinsick modern world cannot be saved from itself by any "wonder drug" or social reform but will have to return to the Bible prescription which treats the whole man and gets at the causes of the disease instead of merely treating the symptoms.

But modern man is not noted for any strong desire to repent and return to the Bible. The majority will probably continue on their way living fast and furiously and trying to desperately repair the damages with some chemical drug, some more aspirins and sleeping pills, or another war to finally "make the world safe once and for all". Dr. James T. Grace, director of the Roswell Park Memorial Institute, noted that the proposed budget of the National Institutes of Health for fiscal 1970 is nearly $20 million less than the previous year's expenditure. The nation, he noted, is spending $127 per person per year to wage the war in Viet Nam, but only 93 cents per person per year for cancer research. As usual, 'civilized man' spends more on killing than on healing. Dr. John H. Knowles, head of Massachusetts General Hospital, in January, 1970 addressed an annual scientific convention and drew sustained applause when questioning America's current priorities: "We are spending twice on the supersonic transport what we spend on medical research in one year, and that's going to cause more disease, more noise, air pollution and traffic congestion. And who ... wants to get to London a few hours earlier anyway?"

INCREASING IATROGENIC DISEASE

Furthermore it seems that every marvelous new "wonder drug" brings with it its lethal side-effects and the incidence of "iatrogenic disease" is tremendously increasing. "Iatrogenic disease" is that caused by doctors, drugs or hospitals and embraces drug shock, antibiotic super-infection, new hospital-raised strains of "staph", serum sickness, vaccinosis, addiction through pain-killers, excessive radiation, malformation of the unborn by experimental drugs (like thalidomide), shot-gun type of over-medication, etc. M. L. Gross in his book, "THE DOCTORS", states: "It might be conservative to estimate death from doctor-caused disease in the magnitude of 200,000 (persons) a year. ... Physicians and modern medicine have thus become a close rival of cancer and heart disease as a major killer of man." (Page 282).

Rather than stubbornly seeking more of the same approach, is it not time to turn back to simpler and safer alternative approaches to modern chemical drugs? This book was written to suggest a new look at the old-fashioned herbal remedies of our forefathers. At the very worst, if they would not help us much, they might not KILL us! At the best, they might prove to be an inexpensive, simple, natural and harmless help in many conditions which resist cure through modern chemical drugs. (For more information on the subject of the Bible and sickness and health, there are two excellent books to be recommended: "NONE OF THESE DISEASES", by S. I. McMillen, Spire Books, Fleming H. Revell Co., 158 pp., 60 cts.; and "THE CHURCH AND HEALING", by Carl J. Scherzer, The Westminster Press, 1950, 272 pp., $4.00). Although the U.S. is the richest country in the world, it ranks 18th in prevention of infant mortality and only 22nd in longevity (TIME, March 30, 1970).

International recognition that modern industrial civilzation is rapidly poisoning its environment has caused a tremendous swing back to interest in natural foods, natural medicines from herbs, and natural instead of artificial ways of living. Public opinion is mobilizing against industries which are poisoning mankind for their own profit with chemical pollution and chemical pesticides and chemical food additives (which embalm food so that even the bugs will not eat it). Some of the latest developments include alarm over the many poisonous and polluting effects of harsh detergent soaps full of phosphates and enzymes. Ask your local health food dealer for a safe, organic substitute for the poisonous detergents! Another important news item is the widespread alarm over poisoning of foods with pesticides. The government is now advising farmers to try to detoxify cows which have been poisoned by pesticide-polluted feeds through the use of two pounds of activated charcoal per cow per day (to eliminate poisons from the intestinal tract) and a small amount of phenobarbital to stimulate flushing out the liver through the urine. We remind our readers that old herbalists used to prescribe purified charcoal for bad cases of poisoning long ago and that there are much better and safer diuretics than phenobarbital to flush out the liver. We strongly urge that you DETOXIFY your own system with natural, herbal medicine and natural foods!

Research continues to be conducted on plant and herbal remendies for cancer and diabetes, with many new discoveries being made.

In Costa Rica, to cure diabetics, herbalists prescribe 3 leaves with bloodsugar lowering action: one cup of tea made from walnut leaves in the morning; one cup of tea made from avocado leaves in the afternoon; one cup of tea made from eucalyptus leaves at night. This regimen is followed until the urine is sugar-free.

The real cure of diabetes is to be sought in the normalizing of the body's natural functions; following a strict, natural diet plus the use of these herbs has helped many: Dandelion root, Cucumber juice, Carrot juice, juice from wild Carrot leaves. Avoid all white sugar and white, refined flour. A new treatment for cancer of the colon, effective in many cases, has been found in extracts from the leaves of the Camptotheca tree (TIME magazine, August 31, 1970). We are convinced that mankind must return to natural, God-given sources for the clue to the healing of modern civilization's poisonous plagues!

WARNING ! The latest research shows that there are two herbs which have some cancer-causing chemical properties: Sassafrass and Krameria Ixina. The latter is used only in the West Indies and contains powerful deposits of tannin -- habitual users develop cancer of the esophagus. Sassafrass has been used medicinally for centuries but recent studies isolated a potentially cancer-causing chemical in it. Habitual use is discouraged. More than 3,000 cancer-causing chemicals are now known to man. Many of them are used as food preservatives and insecticides. Be cautious -- eat only fresh foods uncontaminated with chemical sprays.

CHAPTER II: Brief History of Various Healing Methods:

"PRIMITIVE" MEDICINE AND THE ANCIENTS

From our modern stand-point, we are accustomed to looking down on most primitive medicine as being a combination of magic and superstition. While much of it was no doubt nonsense, more of it was developed out of trial and error methods until something was found that WORKED and thus was a product of common sense. For example, a fantastic concoction of toad skins was used by some ancient peoples as a treatment for dropsy. Today we know that toad skins are rich in buffagin (which stimulates a free flow of urine and thus helps drain the tissues) and in adrenalin (which speeds heart action, increases blood pressure and speeds excretion of sugar). Thus the primitives were only using common sense in using toad skins — unwittingly they were applying the very elements which could alleviate the dropsy. This has remained throughout history a good test of any healing method: DOES IT WORK? If the method used does not alleviate suffering, it eventually becomes a casualty of history and is discarded. Today many modern drug companies are sending specially trained drug detectives all over the world to collect plants, medicines and cures used by various primitive peoples, in order to analyse them in the laboratory and discover what beneficial elements they might contain.

The ancient Egyptians, despite many foolish superstitions, also had trained physicians who treated illness with drugs, herbs, fumigation, medicated baths, hypnosis, hot or cold water, massage, purgations and surgery. The ancient Mesopotamians codified laws to protect public health and regulate the responsibility of physicians to their patients. Their physicians used surgery, psychology, and numerous remedies or prescriptions compounded from herbs (garlic, onion, leek, dates, cypress, pine, tamarisk, laurel, mandrake, opium, hemp, etc.), from animal substances, and from minerals (sulfur, arsenic, saltpeter, antimony, iron oxide, mercury, alum, naptha, calcined lime etc.). The ancient Chinese physicians had highly specialised methods of diagnosis (recognizing 200 types of pulse, 37 shades of tongue) and treatments included physical exercise, special diets, acupuncture (treating nerve centers with needles), moxibustion, vaccination, and above all herbal medicines (which included 2,000 substances, some of which were ephedrine, chaulmoogra, camphor, opium, etc.). Ancient Hindu therapy was based on hygiene, diet and eliminatory measures; surgery was highly developed, hypnosis was used for anesthesia, vaccination was practised, and many medicinal herbs were in use (such as the even now popular tranquilizer reserpine —used by the Hindus for 30 centuries as a calmant and sedative before modern medicine "discovered" it in 1952!). Really, as the Bible says, there is nothing new under the sun!

ANCIENT GREEK, ROMAN AND EARLY CHRISTIAN
MEDICINE

Healing and religion were conceived of as identical by the Ancient Greeks and Romans. Greek temples dedicated to Aesculapius, god of healing, were actually hospitals built in healthful rural settings, usually with mineral springs at hand, and equipped with bathing pools, gymnasia for exercises, and gardens. Patients underwent purification by fasting, special baths, and fumigations. Then they were treated to relaxing massages, soothing music and hypnotic-suggestions, plus sedatives to induce a drugged sleep in which dreams were supposed to reveal to them the cause of their illness after which the priest-doctors would give them further appropriate treatment. Thousands were healed and in gratitude dedicated offerings to the temples, often gold or silver models of the part of the body which had been diseased and was healed. (This was the ancient origin of the practise found in Catholic shrines of hanging up model parts of the body supposedly healed by miraculous intervention). One of the god Aesculapius' daughters was known as Hygieia (from which we get the name hygiene today) and the other was known as Panakeia, goddess of the healing power found in herbs. To this day the word panacea is still defined as a remedy for almost any disease. These two elements, hygiene and herbal medication summed up the major methods of Greek temple medicine. (Modern doctors still use the Greek staff and serpent symbol and write RX on their prescription — originally a dedication swearing loyalty to the pagan god Jupiter).

Later Greek medical men developed a more empirical (and less psycho-therapeutic) approach. Chief among them was a man named Hippocrates, who has become known as the 'father of modern medicine'. He emphasized the natural causes and natural cures of disease, ceasing to regard the sick as sinners (but regarding sinners as sick). He theorized that sickness was the result more often than not of disobedience of natural laws rather than the result of the gods' anger. His therapy focussed on symptoms rather than dreams and he was careful to make detailed case histories of the patients in order to diagnose the illness. He believed the body possessed its own means of recovery which should be helped with anything that could assist the curative powers of nature. Therapy included exercise, massage, baths, diet, herbs, and drugs. Hippocrates wrote much and created in his famous Oath the standard for professional behavior among doctors (promising to poison nobody, cause no abortions, tell no secrets, remain pure, take care of the poor, provide free instruction for the children of those who taught him medicine, etc.). Skilled herbalists, medical botanists, surgeons and other specialists developed among the Hippocratic doctors.

Roman medical practise was an outgrowth of the Greek and at first most of the physicians were Greek slaves. Gradually medicine was regarded as an honorable calling, medical licenses were required, public health inspected, aqueducts and drainage regulated, medical insurance instituted, antimalarial measures taken, etc. The Romans were especially fond of hydrotherapy or healing methods using water (hot baths, cold baths, steam baths, mineral baths, etc.). However, eventually personal hygiene degenerated into an end instead of a means; physical exercises evolved into a carnival of venal sports, rest into torpid siestas in the shady atrium, and hydrotherapy into effeminate dallying and depravity all day long in the public baths. Wherever the Romans went, they built baths — one such covered twenty acres and included reading rooms, auditoria for lectures, running tracks, covered walks, planted gardens, vaulted ceilings, steam rooms, gaming rooms, swimming pools and gymnasia, with subterranean central heating! The most famous Roman physician was Galen whose therapy included sunshine, warmth, baths, diets, liquids, fasting, rest, anesthesia, operations, and an extensive *materia medica* which included 540 herbs, 180 animal and 100 mineral substances, from which he compounded the famous herbal "galenicals" or vegetable simples. He was an authority on baths and gymnastics and produced 500 writings on every aspect of medical science and practise. As there were few apothecaries, most Roman physicians used mortars to prepare their own medicines, usually of herbs from abounding gardens.

When Christianity came on the scene, it adopted whatever natural healing methods were at hand from Greek and Roman tradition (Luke — one of the Gospel writers— was a Greek physician and undoubtedly continued to dedicate to God's service his skills and talents and knowledge). In addition Christianity made use of the Hebraic code of hygiene and employed much prayer and laying on of hands and anointing with oil in supernatural healing. Jesus Christ set the example for His followers in His concern for the sick and suffering, and commanded His disciples to preach (Mt. 10:7), teach (Mt. 28:19-20), and heal (Mt. 10:1). Christ's spirit of compassion animated His followers to care for the sick, the orphans, the widows, the poor, the hungry, and the helpless.

Care of the sick and poor became a special concern of the Christian diaconate (deacons). It was not long until there were also deaconnesses (Rom. 16:1,2). Although Phebe is the first one mentioned as such in the New Testament, the office may be said to have been in existence during Christ's ministry — women disciples followed Jesus also and "ministered unto Him of their substance" (Luke 8:3). Also see I Timothy 5:3-16. Pliny in his letter to Trajan mentioned them about 110 A.D. when he referred to "young women who are called ministrae (deaconnesses)". As the church grew, these helpers became something like regular nursing orders. It was a deaconess, Fabiola, who founded the first charity hospital at Rome about A.D. 300. She sold her large property and turned it into funds to found an infirmary for the poor and sick. These Christian women served and fed the sick, nursed them, washed their feet and bathed them, clothed them and witnessed to them of Christ's healing power. They developed what was known as the xenodochium, a center of relief and forerunner of the modern hospital. All who needed help were welcome there; bread was distributed (and clothing) to the poor, rooms were set aside for the sick and physicians were stationed there to give free treatment. Money was donated by wealthy converts and members for the upkeep of these places.

The early Christians specialized in such healing practises as prayer, anointing with oil, laying on of hands, the cure of souls (what we would call psycho-therapy) by casting out evil spirits and by pastoral counselling, confession and forgiveness of sins, etc. However, they did not neglect to continue the natural therapies of antiquity. Shops around this time began to sell the wares of the 'rhizopodist', a man who gathered roots and herbs for medicinal purposes. A physician of the Romans named Dioscorides wrote an encyclopedia of herbal medicines called a MATERIA MEDICA, in which he classified some 600 plants, herbs, roots and plant products. (About 90 of them are still in common use in modern medicine). The man of that time who influenced the church in its relation to healing practises more than any other medical man was Pliny, who lived about the time of the last of the apostles. His works were acceptable to the Christians even though he was not a Christian himself. He believed that every plant and herb had some special medicinal value. For every disease there was a plant to cure it, and it was the physician's business to find the right plant. The Christians believed that everything on earth has a value or a purpose, so they accepted Pliny's theory of medicine and his works were in great favor among them.

Galen was also accepted as a medical authority by the Christians; he sought to prescribe the proper herbs to balance the diseased condition. If a person suffered a fever, he favored treating them with a cold (or refrigerant) medicine (such as cucumber seeds). He classified all plants into four types: hot, cold, wet, and dry, to be properly prescribed according to the ailment. The church also used surgery, oils, fruits, leaves, and many other medicines and methods accompanied by prayer to bless or sanctify them.

DURING THE DARK AGES:

During the Dark Ages, it was generally forgotten to practise surgery with antiseptics (such as alcoholic wine or iodine from sea-weed) and so many patients died that surgery fell into disrepute and was left to barbers to practise (together with teeth-pulling and blood-letting). During the Dark Ages religion itself fell into low and ignorant superstitions and all the medical arts declined. Many continued to use local herbs and plants that had stood the test of time but much was forgotten. Several terrible plagues were somewhat alleviated by the churches demanding the observance of Mosaic rules of public hygiene and quarantine but in general ignorance and superstition prevailed with people turning to trust in various relics and charms instead of using sensible medicines and therapies.

PIONEERS AND PLAIN PEOPLE

With the Reformation and Renaissance, from 1517 to 1630, there was a return to rediscovering what the Bible and the ancients had recorded about medicines and healing. A prominent Renaissance physician was Paracelsus, devoted to studying the book of Nature and favoring use of simple natural medicaments. Most highly trained physicians were available only for the rich and the common people had to continue to rely on simple natural therapies. But Paracelsus was known to the Hutterites, a church of simple, Bible-believing Christians who held all property in common and rejected participation in politics and warfare, living quiet, rural lives. Their bonesetters, mid-wives, and herbalists studied the medical treatises of antiquity and in their colonies they offered medicinal baths and other natural therapy treatments which caused the sick to come from far and near to be cured. Other peaceful Plain People, like the Amish and Mennonites, fleeing persecution in Europe, brought with them to America a quiet, sane rural life and simple natural remedies. In America they learned much from the herbal science of the Indians and were able to save many lives that would have been destroyed by the medical superstition of the more "learned" doctors. As Dr. Clive M. McKay of Cornell University has said: "If I had been sick 200 years ago, I would have been better off in the hands of a medicine man of the American Indians than I would have been in those of a European physician. The Indian would have given me mental therapy, food and herb remedies. The European physician would have drained away my blood!" To this day the Pennsylvania Dutch are generally more conversant with herbal home remedies than the sophisticated urban population of American. Pioneer living required that men seek their medicines in field and forest rather than the drugstore. It is an interesting fact that other Plain People, the Shakers, pioneered in mass production of herbs and by 1857 were selling 75 tons of medicinal plants in one season, becoming the first reputable manufacturing druggists in America.

MEDICINE IN MODERN TIMES

Modern times have seen many important discoveries and advances in the medical arts. Chief among them might be mentioned the revelation of human anatomy by Vesalius, the humane approach to surgery by Paré, the discovery of the microscope by Leeuwenhoek, William Harvey's discovery of the circulation of the blood, Louis Pasteur's contribution to the germ theory of disease, etc. Others are now working in biochemistry, atomic physics, ultrasound surgery, immunobiology, psycho-biology, etc. Not only is progress being made in new directions but there is an increasingly humble desire to re-investigate the vital ingredients of herbal medicines used by the ancients and the primitives. There has been a return to dialogue with the patient, the method used by the ancient Assyrians and Greeks, to try to establish a true diagnosis of the disease. Karl Jaspers has defined three main groups of diseases by labelling them somatoses (organic diseases), bioses (functional diseases), and psychoses (psychogenic diseases). But the most modern thinking tends to blur even these distinctions and re-emphasize the ancient and Biblical insights into the intimate connections between physical disease and mental disease with the whole concept of psychosomatic disease. And modern medicine seems to have come full circle in its return, for example, to tranquilizers made from Rauwolfia (snakeroot), an herbal remedy known to the Hindus for 30 centuries! Forty years ago, medical doctors would have laughed to scorn any suggestion that people could have been treated for nervous breakdowns by chewing snakeroot! But now they accept without batting an eye-lash the reserpine extracted from snakeroot for that purpose, plus a thousand other medicinal plant extracts and the pharmaceutical houses are constantly searching for more.

It is a good sign that modern science is recovering enough humility to turn back and search for effective medicines in the place where God said long ago He had put them — in herbs. Why be so wary then of telling the sick about the various herbs that God has caused to grow for the benefit and healing of mankind?

(For more information on the subject of the history of medicine, the following books are interesting: "THE EPIC OF MEDICINE", Ed. by Felix Marti Ibañez, Bramhall House, N.Y., 1962, 294 pp. "THE ASTONISHING HISTORY OF THE MEDICAL PROFESSION", by E. S. Turner, Ballantine Books, N.Y. 1961, 255 pp. "FROM MEDICINE MAN to FREUD", by Jan Ehrenwald, Dell Publishing Co., N.Y., 1956, 416 pp.).

Dr. Lester L. Coleman, a medical columnist writing of hopeful news in medicine, rightly remarks that even the most sophisticated modern physician recognizes that many drugs have been used without our scientific knowledge in tribal areas for many centuries. Tribes that never have wandered out of the wilderness have used herbs and plants by trial and error with great success. Our own so-called modern civilization developed chemical drugs derived from the plants used by so-called "primitives". We wonder, when we consider the hostility and aggression that flourish in our so-called "civilized society", just which society is more primitive! The valuable drug reserpine, for example, so useful in reducing high blood pressure, etc., is only one of many borrowed from the medicine chest of the primitives. Now another tribal plant, Tylophora indica (or Country Ipecacuanha), seems to be a very special blessing for "civilized" patients who have severe allergies and asthma. At a recent meeting of the American Academy of Allergy, Dr. D. M. Shizpuri of the University of New Delhi said that he knew of no modern drug which was able to suppress the symptoms of hayfever, nasal allergy and asthma for as long as three months, as does a single leaf of the Tylophora indica plant when given to patients every day for a week. The relief given to asthma sufferers was tremendous and modern medical science has been urged to study this plant.

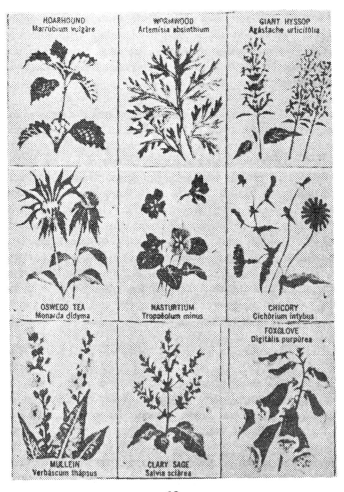

CHAPTER III: Brief Summary of Useful Methods of Natural Healing:

In what we have already briefly reviewed about the history of medicine's various healing methods, we have remarked on the danger of any one-sided, extremist approach to the healing arts. Doctors, like any other professional men, are seen throughout history to be tempted with establishing their own status and security at the expense of organized intolerance towards other kinds of medical practitioners who might use differing methods (and perhaps therefore be thought of as "competitors"). But if we accept the basic truth that it is really Nature which accomplishes true healing under God's sovereignty, then we are able to become more open to any useful method of natural healing whether or not it is recognized, promoted, organized and admired by the prevailing orthodox medical association or not. History shows us repeatedly how important discoveries in medicine were ridiculed, persecuted and slandered by organized, orthodox medical guilds or trade unions (who adopted a kind of monopolistic attitude toward healing, damning anything that did not adjust itself to prevailing theories and fads). It is said of the famous Renaissance doctor Paracelsus, "He was called a quack, an impostor, because he cured sick folks by unaccustomed methods." Such fanatical intolerance is unfortunate.

Paracelsus was born near Zurich, Switzerland, and became an itinerant physician, studying the book of nature. He bequeathed to medicine a dynamic pathology explaining disease as a weakening of the vital principle and his therapy was based on the curative power of nature, believing each malady to have its specific remedy in the surrounding world. He favored simple medicaments and introduced into therapy metals, tinctures, and essences, making him the forerunner of medical bio-chemistry. Any sensible view of medicine realizes that the human body as originally created by God from the "dust of the earth", must naturally contain a spectrum of the numerous elements in nature (sometimes only in very minute, trace element form). The body lacking such natural elements in balance is bound to suffer deficiency and disease. Natural healing methods will aim at replenishing and restoring the missing elements and crippled functions and eliminating the toxic wastes and imbalances.

"DOTH NOT NATURE ITSELF TEACH YOU?"

It stands to reason that the best source of natural restoratives will be the things of nature itself: natural sunlight, natural pure water and juices for drinking, natural foods without dangerous artificial additives, natural herbal medicines instead of dangerous artificial drugs, natural exercise, etc. God has stored in the treasure house of nature all that is necessary for the health of the human body. It should be the function of the medical arts to study nature and apply its secrets. Besides the Book of Nature, God has also blessed mankind with the Book of the Bible which addresses itself to the healing of soul and spirit. That cannot be worthy of the name of true medical art which does not address itself to the study and cure of body, soul and spirit by God-given natural (and supernatural) methods. Before proceeding further, we will survey here the various useful types of natural healing methods practised throughout the ages. "The Lord hath created medicines out of the earth, and he that is wise will not abhor them." (Ecclesiasticus 38:4). "Doth not even nature itself teach you?" (I. Corinthians 11:14).

NATURAL MEDICINES SAFER

If one is not to adopt any extremist view which arbitrarily excludes or discards any medical treatment on the mere basis of prejudice, then one will be open to a versatile approach which might include any beneficial method. Alas, some medical schools of thought often tend to be like the more fanatical religious sects — each supposes itself the sole possessor of the whole truth and automatically condemns all others as absolute charlatans and heretics. Such is the many-sidedness of human nature, body, soul and spirit, that some complicated ailments may only respond to a specialised medical method and one should be open to the use of whatever is naturally appropriate. Yet those methods which are the most artificial and the farthest removed from the natural tend to be the most dangerous. It has been definitely proven, for example, that there are chemical cancer-producing agents and one must be quite stubbornly blind not to see any connection between the increasing use of powerful cancer-producing chemicals, insecticides and food additives, tobacco use, industrial air-pollutions and the enormous corresponding increase of cancer in modern urban society. This inclines the natural healing practitioner towards a "drugless therapy" which shuns powerful synthetic drugs. It stands again to reason that natural herbal medicines can be more easily assimilated than powerful artificial drugs with unknown and perhaps degenerative side-effects. It was Hippocrates, the 'father of medicine', who said: "If anyone believes medical art capable of performing more than nature allows, he is either mad or ignorant."

It must also be borne in mind that there are two basic approaches to all medicine —that which is primarily curative (treating the symptoms of the disease after its onset), and that which is primarily preventive (treating the prospective patient to instruction and methods aimed at preventing the onset of the disease). One need not be sick in order to learn the principles of healthful living! Following a brief outline of orthodox medical science, we shall discuss some methods of natural healing which have been employed throughout history, in both ancient and modern cultures. A balanced approach to medical arts would not reject any of these methods *a priori*, but be willing to choose from the best and most useful of all of them.

ALLOPATHY (Orthodox Medical Science)

This is the approach followed by the vast majority of licensed medical doctors practising in modern industrial nations. It relies increasingly nowadays on three tactics: first, general practitioners diagnose simple ailments, perform minor surgery and dispense popular prescription drugs prepackaged by the great pharmaceutical firms; secondly, discovery of common functional ailments and referral to hospitalization, orthopedia and surgery for correction; thirdly, suspicion or discovery of some more complicated disorder and subsequent referral to a specialist in that area (such as an obstetrician, orthopedist, psychiatrist, allergist, pediatrician, heart specialist, eye specialist, etc). While this system of medical treatment does much good and is the most popular and common, it has definite limitations and weaknesses and the patient should learn to exercise all due CAUTION especially in the area of these abuses: 1—the danger of unnecessary surgery undertaken primarily for the profit motive (this has been documented and proven over and over again that unscrupulous doctors order unnecessary operations); 2— the danger of overpaying and exorbitant fees through the common practise of one doctor receiving a kick-back payment from the specialist to whom he has referred you (for example, the doctor refers patients to another doctor for 25% or 35% of the fee charged); 3—the danger of the patient overpaying for medicine when the doctor prescribes it by its famous brand-name instead of by its generic or medicinal-contents name and this will be a difference sometimes in paying 5 or 10 times more for the SAME medicine (your doctor may be ignorant of the fact that his PHYSICIAN'S DESK REFERENCE list of drugs is actually an advertising book framed by the commercial interests of the pharmaceutical industry, or he may even be getting a kick-back from the druggist for prescribing the more expensive brands); 4—the danger of iatrogenic disease or complications brought on the patient by the doctors, the hospitals or the powerful synthetic drugs used (this is becoming so common that increasingly victimized patients or their survivors are fighting back by suing the doctors, hospitals and drug companies; the January 19, 1970 NEWSWEEK states that from 6,000 to 9,000 malpractice suits are being brought each year and the American Medical Association estimated that one in seven U.S. doctors has been sued at least once). Incompetent doctors can no longer bury their "mistakes" with impunity —nowadays the widow often returns directly from the burial to consult an attorney!

To help the potential patient understand these dangers, it is useful to read three books previously mentioned: "THE HEALERS", by Anonymous M.D. (Putnam), written by a medical doctor who feared to use his own name or he would be persecuted by his colleagues — he documents case after case of doctor malpractice, profiteering, incompetence, venality, unnecessary operations and murder: "THE DOCTORS", by Martin L. Gross (Dell); and "THE AMERICAN HEALTH SCANDAL", by Roul Tunley (Dell), which documents the poor medical attention Americans receive compared with many other, smaller nations of the world. These are well-documented, reasonably written books which can help to alert the public to be CAUTIOUS when it comes to treatment by regular, licensed medical doctors, as well as being cautious about quacks who promise fantastic cures (at fantastic prices). Also helpful are these additional books: "THE HANDBOOK OF PRESCRIPTION DRUGS", by Richard Burack, M.D., Pantheon Books, Random House, N.Y., 1967, $1.95, 191 pp. (which explains how you can get your prescription drugs by their generic names and avoid the racket of paying many times more for the same thing under a famous brand name). For example, for the same anti-malarial medicine (Chloroquine Phosphate), you can buy 100 tablets for $2.80 or you can pay as high as $6.70 for the SAME THING under a "better brand name"! Or take another drug, Erythromycin, which is given to save people from dying from allergic reactions to penicillin — yet you may get jaundice from taking it! Or, you could buy 1,000 tablets of Digitalis (.1 gm. tablets) for as little as $1.36 or you can pay $18.50 for the SAME THING, if you are not aware of the brand names racket. Also consult, "WHAT YOU SHOULD KNOW ABOUT PILLS", by Robert A. Liston, Pocket Books, N.Y., 1968, 160 pp., 95 cts.; "THE SHOCKING HISTORY OF DRUGS", by Richard Bathison, Ballantine Books, 1968, 50 cts., 254 pp.; or "SUPER DRUG STORY", by Morris A. Bealle, Columbia Publishing Co., 1968, 250 pp. Should there come a time when surgery is absolutely necessary (—be sure to consult several doctors independently to verify that a REAL need exists or that there may not be a less radical way of correcting the condition), a very helpful book to read is, "UNDERSTANDING SURGERY", by Dr. Robert E. Rothenberg, Pocket Books, 1968, 95 cts., 717 pp.

NATUROPATHY (Natural Medical Arts):

This is an approach to medical treatment that includes a wide range of natural methods that have been used in one form or another throughout the centuries, such as Dietetics, Physiotherapy, Hydrotherapy, Chiropractic, Homeopathy, Herbal Therapy, Neuropractic, etc. The one single thing that differentiates these techniques of naturopathy from the methods of allopathy is that they are generally so simple that even a layman can grasp their principles and practise them in a rudimentary way as first aid or a home remedy for his own benefit. This is not to say that they are not based on considerable science, research and the vast experience of the human race over the centuries, but it is a fact that like the Bible principles of cleanliness, rest, purity and temperance, they are easily understood, often passed on from one generation to another by tradition, but seldom practised fully without real dedication. People easily perceive that they make common sense but their conscientious practise requires diligence and perseverance and therefore they are quickly rejected by the self-indulgent and lazy who prefer any medicine which offers them a quick pill, a shot, or a sudden operation instead of a life-long regimen of safe and sane temperance.

Naturopathic, homeopathic and herbal therapists emphasize prevention for maintenance of natural health. They regulate the diet and habits of living on a natural basis, promote elimination, teach correct breathing and wholesome exercises, adjust and correct mechanical faults in the spine and other bone structures, work to establish the right mental and emotional attitudes, and insofar as they succeed in doing this, they build health and diminish the possibility of disease. Naturopaths do not deny the necessity of combatting germs, bacterial infections, parasites and other diseases that invade the body but they emphasize more building up body defenses against all disease through natural preventive measures.

As in the case of allopathy, so too naturopathy is subject to abuses on the part of some unscrupulous practitioners who aim more for pecuniary profit than for healing. A danger sign is always when some promoter begins to tout only one minor approach or patented medicine or packaged "health food" as a kind of magic cure-all, and neglects or discards all the numerous, sensible healing disciplines in order to advertise and sell his own "one-shot" patented gimmick. An amusing yet stimulating book of warning along this line is "THE NUTS AMONG THE BERRIES", (An Expose of America's Food Fads), by Ronald M. Deutsch, Ballantine Books, N.Y., 1967, 320 pp., 95 cts. Beware of any "miracle cancer cures", for example; many skin cancers can be treated successfully by herbal medicines but few if any medicines exist capable of successfully treating an internal cancer which has gone into metastasis (the spreading of the cancer from its original starting point throughout the body by the lymph system, etc.). A cancer reaching that stage is usually curable only by a miracle, so if some promoter comes along and offers to cure the most desperate cancerous conditions with magic pills costing $200 apiece, suspect a charlatan. Unscrupulous promoters in any health field try to take some small fragment of truth and magnify it into a money-making cure-all. For a time it becomes a fad or even a cult but finally dies out.

The prevention of cancer seems to be the only practical way of dealing with it. But prevention of cancer involves a regime of life few people will adopt. Avoidance of cancer-causatives (carcinogenics) must be practised, including such things as air and water pollution, pesticides, overcooking, excesses of fats and sugars, X-rays, soot, petroleum products, smoke, fumes, radiation, cigarette smoking, food dyes, chemical food additives and flavorings, eating and drinking of very hot foods and even wrong or negative emotions! Emotional states conducive to cancer include anger, resentment, hatred, fear, jealousy and greed. The Bible says, for example "Ye rich men,... Your gold and silver is CANCEROUS,... and shall eat your flesh as it were fire (James 5:1,3)." Here it is not a case of what you eat but of what eats you! Another reputed cause of cancer is sluggishness of the lymphatic circulation either locally or generally, from faulty and excessive nutrition, lack of exercise and wrong living in general. Helpful herbs in cancer treatment have been especially those containing potassium, iron and other vital minerals usually deficient in these cases, such as Grapes, Red clover flowers, Violet leaves, Docks, Red beet juice, etc. Growing in the jungles of Costa Rica is a milk weed plant Indians have used for ages as a remedy for cancer, warts and similar growths, called the cancerillo plant. But no single treatment has proved always effective since cancer is not a single disease but the terminal sympton of several diseases.

Any fairly intelligent and sensible person ought to realize that there is no magic cure-all that can be neatly rolled up into one pill or shot yet there are millions of people constantly seeking such a magic potion. This is what provides a following for the various fads and cults of pseudo-medicine. It might be taken as a matter of fact that the doctor never cures a disease; he ennables the body to cure itself by assisting it in its struggle. Following is a brief outline of the naturopathic methods that have been found helpful throughout the ages. Since this book is primarly devoted to a survey of herbal therapy, we can do no more than mention these other medical arts in passing and refer the reader to suitable books for further study.

DIETETICS (Food Therapy):

Proper food is probably the single most important organic factor in maintaining health and curing disease. It is widely recognized nowadays that deficiency in the minerals and vitamins, proteins and carbohydrates, or intoxication from overeating, or from eating of artificial, devitalized or poisoned foods, is a major cause of disease and death. Millions are literally digging their graves with their teeth and committing suicide with knife and fork! A few helpful books on this vital subject are: "OUR DAILY POISON", by Leonard Wickenden (Davin-Adair Co., 1956, 189 pp.); "THE LEGACY OF DOCTOR WILEY", by Maurice Natenberg (Regent House, Chicago, 1957, 166 pp.); "THE NATIONAL MALNUTRITION", by D. T. Quigley (Lee Foundation, 1943, 113 pp.); "FOOD IS YOUR BEST MEDICINE", by Henry G. Bieler (Random House, N. Y., 1965, 236 pp.); "LET'S EAT RIGHT TO KEEP FIT", by Adelle Davis (Harcourt, Brace, World Co., 1954, 322 pp.); "NUTRITION FOR HEALTH", by Dr. Alice Chase (Parker Publ. Co., 1954, 319 pp.); "HELPING YOUR HEALTH WITH ENZYMES", by

Carlson Wade (Parker Publ. Co., 1966, 224 pp.); "CALORIES, VITA-
MINS AND COMMON SENSE", by H. Curtis Wood, Jr. (Belmont
Books, 1962, 125 pp.); "THE GRAPE CURE", by Johanna Brandt
(St. Marks Printing Corporation, 1956, 192 pp.). Food therapy is a
field in which there are many fads so it is well to keep in mind that
only nature can produce natural vitamins and no exorbitantly priced and
highly advertised "health food" or "food supplement" can be as healthful
as the simple foods organically grown in your own garden. This is an
area in which even the government is taking increasing concern over
suspect food additives and indiscriminate poisoning of foods by insecticides such as D.D.T. There is no substitute for a balanced diet.

POMOTHERAPY   (Live Food Juices Therapy):

Since the body itself is more than 90% water in composition and
the life of the body is carried by the blood stream, it has been recognized
for centuries that one's health is largely dependent on what one drinks
(or fails to drink). Much disease is caused by toxic wastes accumulating
in the body for want of being flushed out with sufficient liquids. Daily
consumption of several pints of pure water, glasses of fresh fruit or vegetable
juices, cups of fragrant herbal teas— these are one's simplest insurance
of inner hygiene. Avoidance of impure or contaminated water, avoidance
of alcoholic beverages, carbonated "soft" drinks, coffee and commercial
tea, etc. are as necessary as avoiding a liquid-starved diet. Thomas De
Schauer has said, "Constipation, indigestion, anemia are all caused more
or less from the deficiency of water in the system". The nicest wedding
present you could give any young couple would be a juicer and a book
on the specific benefits of the various live food juices. For further study:
"KNEIPP HERBS", by Dr. Benedict Lust (96 pp.); "RAW JUICE
THERAPY", by John B. Lust; NATURAL METHOD OF HEALING
YOUR KIDNEY TROUBLES", by B. Lust (80 pp.); "RAW VEGE-
TABLE JUICES", by N. W. Walker (127 pp.); "THE MIRACLE
OF FRESH, RAW JUICES", by D. R. Hiatt (40 pp.); "DRINK YOUR
TROUBLES AWAY", by John Lust (182 pp.); "LIVE FOOD JUI-
CES", by H. E. Kirschner (120 pp.); "SALUD POR JUGOS", by
Carlos Kozel (48 pp. in Spanish).

NESTEIATHERAPY   (Fasting Therapy):

It has been said that fasting is as old as life. Nature provided both
feasts and famine to maintain the vital balance and a modern economy of
gluttony and superabundance can kill more widely and insidiously than any
famine in nature. Nearly all the religions made ample use of the practise
of fasting; in the Bible, fasting is frequently mentioned in conjunction with
prayer for the purpose of counter-acting self-indulgence and strengthening

of spiritual power. Fasting as a therapeutic healing device has been frequently employed. The following books will suggest helpful methods of controlled, therapeutic fasting. Be sure to fast only under a doctor's care and careful observation if you are planning for an extensive fast. Many a seemingly "hopeless case" has recovered under the regimen of a controlled fast to eliminate the toxins. (For further study, see: "THE HEALTH SECRETS OF A NATUROPATHIC DOCTOR", by M. O. Garten, Parker Publ. Co., 1967, 238 pp.; "THE NATURAL WAY TO HEALTH THROUGH CONTROLLED FASTING", by Carlson Wade, Parker Publ. Col., 1968, 206 pp.; "ABOUT SCIENTIFIC FASTING", by Linda B. Hazard, B. Lust Publ., 1969, 64 pp.; "THE PROCESS OF PHYSICAL PURIFICATION THROUGH THE NEW AND EASY WAY TO FAST", by Dr. Teofilo De La Torre, Publ. in Costa Rica; "THE NO BREAKFAST PLAN AND THE FASTING CURE", by Edward H. Dewey, Health Culture Co., 207 pp., 1900).

HYPNOTHERAPY (Sleep Therapy):

Sleep therapy has been widely used by the ancients, not only in hypnotic trances and drug-induced trances, but even in more simple prescriptions for prolonged rest and normal sleep. Modern times have seen the "rediscovery" of these ancient methods including putting of patients in prolonged "deep sleep" to allow body recuperation. It is a truism that if we do not observe regular hours of rest and relaxation, to come apart for a time of prayer and meditation, relaxation and recreation, then tension causes us to "come apart" in pieces by a disastrous breakdown. Man's little life is bounded with sleep, as Shakespeare said, and we spend a third of our lives in bed, but normal, relaxed sleep is nonetheless a healing therapy for the mind and body. Numerous simple herbs exist which help facilitate relaxing sleep without recourse to habit forming drugs. The quickest short-cut to nervous break-down is cheating on sleep. Communist and other types of dictatorships practise brain-washing captives by continuously depriving them of sleep until they break-down and then re-mold their shattered thinking with propaganda. In Latin America a brief afternoon nap or siesta is found to be a good protection against the harsh noon sun of the tropics.

HYDROTHERAPY (Bath Therapy):

Sometimes called "balneotherapy", bath therapy employs techniques used in the healing arts for thousands of years. Steam baths, mineral baths, sweat baths, hot or cold baths, showers, douches, enemas, colonic and intestinal irrigations, sitz baths, compresses — all have their valid uses in eliminating wastes and stimulating restoration. Baths using infusion of aromatic herbs and oils will be discussed later in the herbal section. It is a truism that cleanliness is next to godliness. For centuries men have enjoyed the curative effects of mineral springs — the constant bathing and drinking of the water keep the bowels and kidneys active and the pores of the skin open — these are the three principal channels for eliminating body wastes and poisons. Each square inch of our skin has 3,500 sweating tubes or perspiration outlets, each one of which acts like a drain tile for removing wastes and impurities from our system. Altogether there are almost 40 miles of these drain tiles in the skin! If you block them, man sickens and dies. Bath therapy to keep these pores open is vital to health.

PNEUMOTHERAPY (Breathing Therapy):

Although breathing therapy has been practised for thousands of years in the Orient (in such arts as yoga), Western medicine is only now discovering how vital this is . A major assist in health can come just from learning how to breathe properly — most people have the bad habit of shallow breathing instead of deep breathing, putting only a portion of the lungs to efficient use. The life-giving oxygen, inhaled and then transferred by the lungs to the blood and thence to all parts of the body can be used as a vehicle of therapy through the inhalation of volatile, aromatic herbal oils as a vapor (see discussion on this in the herbal section). The great crime of modern industrial civilization is its air pollution and cigarette promotion, poisoning the lungs of the city man. A recent scientific survey revealed that technically the last clean air in the U.S. disappeared six years ago! Polluted air is defined as 2,000 particles of pollution in a section of air half the size of a sugar cube; most city areas today average 15,000 particles and this is growing at the rate of 1,500 per year! Pollution level is fatal for human beings at 35,000 particles and this level will be reached in the U. S. by the 1980's! To survive, mankind may have to cover the cities with domes and wear masks, or move to pioneer countries that are underdeveloped, OR DIE. Several stimulating books on this subject are: "WITH EVERY BREATH YOU TAKE", by Howard R. Lewis (Crown Publishers, N. Y., 1965, 333 pp.); "CANCER BY THE CARTON", by S. I. McMillen (Fleming Revell Co., 1963, 63 pp.); "SILENT SPRING", by Rachel Carson (Houghton Mifflin Co., 1962, 368 pp.). Mankind is drowning in his own poisons. Man must take action to stop polluting the environment and learn to protect and purify his breathing. Also see the "Consumer's Union Report on Smoking" (1963, 222 pp.); "OUR PLUNDERED PLANET", by Fairfield Osborn (Pyramid Books, 1968, 176 pp.); and "ANIMAL MACHINES - AN EXPOSE OF FACTORY FARMING", by Ruth Harrison, Ballantine Books, 1966, 220 pp.

MECHANOTHERAPY (Corrective Massage and Adjustment):

Under this general heading would come such therapies as osteopathy, chiropractic, neprapathy, neuropractic and the various systems of massage and body manipulation which try to correct faults and lesions in the bony structure, musculature, and neural channels. Among the many books available on these therapies, you might read "YOUR HEALTH AND CHIRO-PRACTIC" by Thorp McClusky (Pyramid Books, 1962, 254 pp.). Many of the ailments of the human body can be cured or ameliorated by physical therapy, that cannot be helped by surgery or drugs. Thomas Alva Edison was so optimistic about the possibilities of physical therapy of this type that he said, "The doctor of the future will give no medicine, but will interest his patients in the care of the human frame, in diet, and in the cause and prevention of disease." The naturopathic doctor freely uses the wonderful world of corrective herbs and foods in conjuction with mechanotherapies, but tends to avoid the use of powerful synthetic drugs. Millions of people in modern society suffer excruciating pain from "back trouble" that could be helped by mechanotherapy.

PHYSIOTHERAPY   (Corrective Gymnastic Exercises) :

This is another much neglected field which is now receiving great attention as it is understood that man's physical health rapidly deteriorates without sensible exercise of the limbs and muscles. New or rediscovered techniques include such therapies as the Chinese Tai-chi Chuan dynamic tension exercises, isometrics, simple eye exercises to lessen the need for glasses, etc. The whole human system suffers when muscle tone is lost. The ancients understood and applied this in gymnastics. Many books outlining exercises are available.

PSYCHOTHERAPY   (Psychological Therapy) :

This is such a vast field one can only mention briefly that all sound medical art must recognize the intimate unity between physical health and mental and spiritual health. Doctors realize that a high percentage of all sicknesses are psychosomatic — having their origin in mental, spiritual and emotional stresses which result in physical disease and death. Loving, understanding counselling and the relief of confession are two universal therapies in the cure of souls. However, this field has its quacks too who try to speak "peace, peace" where there is no peace. Further stimulating reading: "A HISTORY OF THE CURE OF SOULS", John T. McNeil (Harper Bros., 1951, 371 pp.); "ANXIETY IN CHRISTIAN EXPERIENCE", by Wayne E. Oates (Westminster Press, 1955, 156 pp.); "THE HISTORY OF PSYCHIATRY", by F. G. Alexander and S. T. Selesnick (Harper & Row, 1966, 471 pp.); "ERRORS OF PSYCHOTHERAPY", by Sebastian De Grazia (Doubleday, 1952, 288 pp.); "THE CASE AGAINST PSYCHO-ANALYSIS", by Andrew Salter (Henry Holt & Co., 1952, 179 pp.). The best book on psychotherapy remains the Bible with its glorious prescription: "Perfect love casts out fear." All the forms of fear (guilt, anxiety, worry, envy, greed, insecurity, hatred) are best treated by the love of God in Christ. Salvation experientially is salvation by God's love from man's destructive and disintegrative fears. The Bible says: "A merry heart doeth good like a medicine." (Proverbs 17:22). Christ died on the cross, shedding His blood as an innocent sacrifice for the guilty; God's healing love and forgiveness speak peace and joy to the troubled heart. What medicine can surpass that?

BIOCHEMICAL THERAPY (Tissue Salt Therapy):

This therapy treats diseases caused by an imbalance or deficiency in twelve vital mineral salts present in the human body. For more information consult: "DR. SCHUESSLER'S BIOCHEMISTRY", by Dr. J. B. Chapman (New Era Laboratories Ltd., London, 1965, 191 pp.). Calcium, iron, phosphorous, sodium, etc. are vital in their proper balance to maintaining or regaining health.

Miscellaneous Therapies:

Numerous other naturopathic therapies are also in use, such as radiotherapy, electrotherapy, diathermy, phototherapy, ultraviolet rays, sunlight or heliotherapy, radiant light, etc.). A sensible person will welcome the proper use of any special therapy which alleviates human suffering, without committing the folly of dogmatically claiming that ONE AND ONLY ONE KIND OF THERAPY IS POSSIBLE. A like kind of folly, only more vicious, is that which claims a monopoly on some therapy for the purpose of making the monopolist rich at the expense of others. The greatest curse in any area of medicine is not merely quackery (of which there is plenty enough) but GREED for inordinate profits. Any sound therapy should be simple, natural and available inexpensively to the poor.

HOMEOPATHY and HERBALISM:

Last of all, and most important of all the naturopathic therapies, modern homeopathy is based on principles of herbalism going back thousands of years to the medicinal botanicals of the ancients. Homeopathy is a method of using natural medicines to treat various diseases and weaknesses on the basis of the natural law that "like cures like". Modern medical science makes use of this same principle in treatment for allergies where a certain medicine is used which in diluted form stimulates the body to set up defenses, immunities or desensitivity against the allergy. Homeopathic medicines are derived from the mineral, animal and vegetable kingdoms but the vast majority come from live plants and herbs and are classified as botanicals. These are made from the whole plant or its parts (such as flowers, roots, seed, bark, twigs, leaves and the juice). These homeopathic medicines are made in various strengths or potencies and prepared according to official and accepted standards. The HOMEOPATHIC PHARMACOPEIA OF THE UNITED STATES was authorized by an act of Congress, has been recognized by the U. S. Government since 1938, and is the official standard for homeopathic prescriptions. Besides hundreds of naturopathic practitioners that use herbal medicines, there are more than a thousand regular medical doctors in the U. S. who have been trained in homeopathic medicine and use it in addition to orthodox medicine. (The directory of these doctors by address and state can be secured from the American Institute of Homeopathy, 2726 Quebec Street, N. W., Washington, D. C. 2008).

Herbalism is the oldest, safest and surest healing art in all the world. Nothing has ever been able to approach nature when it comes to healing and nature's way is through plants and herbs of the good earth. Encyclopedias of herbal remedies existed among the ancient Egyptians, Assyrians, Greeks, Romans, Hindus and Chinese. The herbalist prescribes proven remedies for specific conditions and nature does the healing. HERBS ARE TRULY FOODS THAT ACT AS MEDICINE. Herbs are nature's food and nature's medicine. Samuel Hahnemann (1755-1843), founder of modern homeopathy, proved by actual research, clinical experience and painstaking observation that the traditional knowledge propounded by the herbalists is correct.

Because homeopathy and herbalism are so natural and simple that any layman can have on hand in his own home the proven remedies, or can purchase them at small cost from homeopathic and herbal suppliers, these healing arts are within the competence of any intelligent layman. But for this same reason these medical arts are hated and slandered by many professional doctors as a species of "Quackery". But who was proven right when nature cure healers had been telling mankind for thousands of years to eat liberally of fresh, unprocessed, vital herbs and foods and their injunctions were ignored and ridiculed by "modern medical science"? Finally the scientists and food specialists got busy and coined the word VITAMIN (which merely means the vital elements in foods)! Nor was this all — when the public became convinced of the value of vitamins, commercial manufacturing interests saw a great chance of making money out of producing synthetic, artificial vitamins (from such delectable garbage as the waste by-products of coal tar, for example)! We should obtain our vitamins as nature itself provides them!

Herbalism and homeopathy were not intended to replace a doctor or healer or to primarily be the authority for each person to prescribe for and treat himself. It only stands to reason that men trained in the healing arts are more qualified to diagnose and properly prescribe. On the other hand, homeopathic and herbal remedies have a unique advantage as they are made up of harmless, natural herbs and permit the discerning individual to analyse his own symptoms and select the remedy for common discomforts and minor indispositions that are not serious enough to warrant wasting the doctor's valuable time. Any illness of a serious nature or which does not respond to treatment should be warrant for calling in the services of a competent professional physician, whether medical doctor or naturopath. Some helpful books for further study: "PROVEN REMEDIES" by J. H. Oliver (Thorsons Publ., 1968, 92pp.); "THE HERBALIST", by Joseph E. Meyer (Indian Botanic Gardens, 1960, 304 pp.); "BACK TO EDEN", by Jethro Kloss (Longview Publishing House, 671 pp.); "USING PLANTS FOR HEALING", by Nelson Coon (Hearthside Press, 1963, 272 pp.); "THE SIMMONITE-CULPEPPER HERBAL REMEDIES" (Foulsham & Co., n.d., 12 pp.); " THE MODERN BOTANIC PRESCRIBER", by E. Powell (Fowler & Co., 1965, 136 pp.); "HOMEOPATHY", by G. W. Boericke (Am. Inst. of Homeopathy, n. d., 23 pp.); "THE LITTLE HOMEOPATHIC PHYSICIAN", by W. Gutman (Boericke & Tafel, 1961, 41 pp.); "SALUD Y CURACION POP YERBAS". by Carlos Kozel, (in Spanish, 1966, 842 pp.); "KNAURS HEILPFLANZENBUCH", by Hugo Hartwig (in German, Droemersche Publ., 1964, 404 pp.)

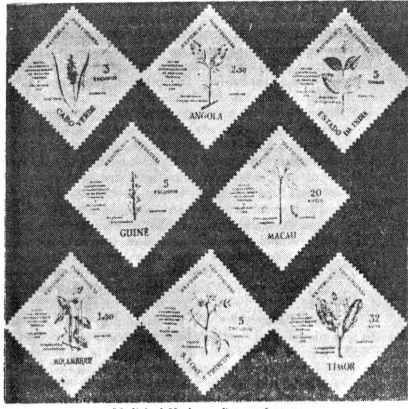

Medicinal Herbs on Postage Stamps

CHAPTER IV: My Own Experience of Healing from an Arthritic Condition by Natural Therapy:

Our family moved from the U. S. to Costa Rica (in Central America) in September of 1968, to do mission work. Although having lived for a time on an island in the Caribbean area before, this was our first experience of moving to the tropics to stay. 38 years old and in general good health at the time we moved down, I was considerably overweight at 205 pounds. We located in an ideal rural area with plenty of sunshine, warm during the day yet cool at night because we are at an altitude of 2,700 feet. My first mistake health-wise was in not realizing I needed much less meat in the tropics than I was used to consuming in the States.

Because delicious steaks and roasts were less than half the cost down here of what we had to pay in the U. S., I soon found myself eating even more meat than formerly. This set me up to overloading my system with fats and uric acid. Besides I was overeating ice cream and neglecting a balanced diet of fruit and vegetables. My good wife remarked several times, "You are practically living on steak and ice cream!" But I did not pay any attention as I was "too busy" to bother with any care in eating a more balanced diet — besides, what could be possibly wrong with good old American-style steak and ice cream?

Soon after this classic framework of bad diet and overwork, I was slightly injured in an automobile accident, receiving a severe blow in my lower back around the area of the kidneys. I got up and walked away from the accident hardly realizing that I was hurt at all but the damage was done. My kidneys, already overloaded by my unbalanced diet, suffered a severe blow, bled internally and became hampered in their functions. It was probably at this time that uric acid began flooding my system and settling in my joints, setting up arthritic symptoms.

Several days after the accident, it got so that I had difficulty walking swiftly; it seemed as if my limbs were freezing up at the joints and I soon could only take shuffling steps. This so alarmed me that I went to a medical doctor for a check-up; when he took a sample of my urine, it was dark red in color (probably from the internal bleeding). The doctor jumped at once to the conclusion that I had contracted hepatitis and even though an immediate lab test for hepatitis proved negative, the doctor insisted I would get it if I did not already have it (!) and gave me a powerful gamma globulin shot (which probably aggravated my already poisoned system).

When night came I woke up with an excruciating pain in my hip and found out I could not even walk anymore. Helped into the car and driven to the hospital, I was given a pain-killing shot in my hip and slept poorly for the rest of the night. Over the next days I was subjected to batteries of blood tests and x-rays and urinalyses, etc. After almost two weeks of hospitalization (during which I returned home for a few days but had to go back because of the terrible joint pain and crippling), I was not improved. My joints were red and inflamed and crippled. My feet and ankles were swollen; my hands and fingers were likewise swollen and painful. Several specialists consulted together on my case but could only tell me that I probably had rheumatoid arthritis and might be a cripple for the rest of my life. They felt there was really no cure but that taking large numbers of aspirin might somewhat alleviate the pain! Another doctor thought I had rheumatic fever and another GUESS was that I might have gout or possibly even serum sickness from the unnecessary shot for hepatitis.

My illness continued for weeks, unimproved, and the pain and crippling began to depress me. After considerable prayer about the matter, we began to try changing my diet as well as my doctor. After reading about juice fasts, I went on a six-day carrot juice diet and began to improve at once. I was recommended to a naturopathic doctor (who was also a trained medical doctor and homeopath). Immediately he put me on strict low-protein diet, high in fruits and vegetables and began treating me with simple herbal medicines to clean out my kidneys and gall bladder. Amazing amounts of toxic wastes began to be eliminated from my body. My weight dropped to 175 pounds and I began to feel wonderfully light and energetic, although the arthritic swellings persisted in my hands, ankles and feet. Sweat baths helped to further cleanse my system.

HEALED BY GOD-GIVEN HERBS

Next my doctor assumed that my system was on the way to recovery and put me on a six day course of homeopathic herbal medicine to counteract the arthritic symptoms. The simple medicine cost only about $1.65 in contrast to the hundreds of dollars I had spent in vain on hospitalization, x-rays, etc. In SIX DAYS all symptoms of arthritis had left me and I was FREE of the terrible crippling curse! You can't imagine how joyful my family and I were in having been privileged to discover such a simple, God-given natural therapy with herbs.

For the interest of our readers in the U. S. who may be afflicted with arthritic and rheumatic conditions (and I understand there are millions of such sufferers), the homeopathic herbal medicine which I was treated with was liquid drops of three herbs, all in the potency of 30, Rhus toxicodendron, Rhododendron, and Bryonia. These have been known as useful aids in the treatment of many kinds of arthritic conditions for many years. Consult your physician who is familiar with naturopathic and homeopathic treatment and enquire if a course of these herbs might not be helpful to you. I took ten drops of each daily for six days. Of course, since arthritis and rheumatism are systemic diseases (affecting the whole system), it is also necessary to treat the whole system with purifying fasts, diet, baths, etc., for lasting results. No doubt there are some arthritic or rheumatoid conditions so far advanced that the joints have become more or less permanently hardened and deformed (calcified). Such conditions do not admit of a quick cure as they have been years in worsening. It certainly would not hurt to try natural therapy as modern medical science admits its own helplessness.

I have come out of this trying experience with this terrible illness with more than one blessing. First I am thankful that the Bible is again proved right in its ancient wisdom when it reminds us that God has given us every herb for a purpose (and its leaf for medicine). Secondly, I have been forcibly reminded again that we cannot abuse our bodies by overloading them with an unbalanced diet and expect not to suffer for it. Thirdly, I have become an enthusiastic advocate of natural methods of therapy: diet, fasting, juices, cleansing of the digestive tract, and the use of simple herbal medicines.

Since my frightful experience, I have made a detailed study of naturopathy and homeopathy and secured more than 100 books on the subject from far and wide as well as taking a correspondence course in it. I recommend to all our readers that you practise moderation and a well-balanced diet lest you too overload your system with toxins and bring on some terrible illness. Millions are committing suicide with knife and fork.

Another result of my experience is that I have applied myself to writing this book about the history and practise of natural healing methods from Bible times down to the present. This has been a thrilling experience, well worth the suffering involved. More than a year has passed now with no recurrence of my arthritic condition.

In the section that follows, I shall list simple herbal recipes I have culled from my reading and experience, that may be of interest to the general reader. Additional reading matter on the subject of arthritis and rheumatism and the natural approach to their treatment can be found in these books:

"THERE IS A CURE FOR ARTHRITIS", by Paavo A. Airola, Parker Publishing Co., Inc., 1968, 200 pp. "VICTORY OVER ARTHRITIS", by Rasmus Alsaker, Health Culture Co., N. Y., 1956, 205 pp. "HOPE FOR THE ARTHRITIC", by Lucrezia Lopez, Benedict Lust Publications, 1956, 23 pp. "RHEUMATISM: ITS CAUSE, AVOIDANCE AND CURE", October, 1963, issue of *FITNESS AND HEALTH FROM HERBS* magazine, England. "THE ENCYCLOPEDIA OF NATURAL HEALTH", by Max Warmbrand, Groton Press, Inc., 1962, 386 pp.

CHAPTER V.—How Ancient Herbs Are Being Rediscovered as Modern Medicines:

What is an HERB? Some dictionaries indicate an herb is any plant (or part of a plant, such as a leaf) which is valued for its medicinal properties, flavor, scent, culinary qualities or value as a dye. From primitive times to the present day man has used such herbs to augment his comfort and well-being. How did man get started looking to herbs for his medicines? There are three simple reasons: 1. The Bible bids man to look to herbs for his medicines; 2. Man could observe the "dumb animals" turning to herbs for healing; 3. By trial and error, man in his hunger found curative herbs.

Concerning the second of the above reasons, Dr. D. C. Jarvis, in his book "FOLK MEDICINE", says: "I have come to marvel at the instinct of animals to make use of natural laws for healing themselves. They know unerringly which herbs will cure what ills. Wild creatures first seek solitude and absolute relaxation, then they rely on the complete remedies of Nature— the medicine in plants and pure air. A bear grubbing for fern roots; a wild turkey compelling her babies in a rainy spell to eat leaves of the spice bush; an animal, bitten by a poisonous snake, confidently chewing snakeroot — all these are typical examples. An animal with fever quickly hunts up an airy, shady place near water, there remaining quiet, eating nothing but drinking often until its health is recovered. On the other hand, an animal bedeviled by rheumatism finds a spot of hot sunlight and lies in it until the misery bakes out."

Only think of how many herbal medicines were discovered historically by "accident" (or trial and error, or "experience")! Seaweed-derived IODINE, an old Polynesian antiseptic, is a staple in our medicine cabinets. The extract from Foxglove leaves known as DIGITALIS was in use for centuries for heart trouble before medical science ever discovered it. SNAKEROOT (Rauwolfia) was used by Hindus as a tranquilizer for 30 centuries before modern medicine discovered it. For centuries old-time Greek shepherds dressed infected wounds with bread mold and only recently a modern scientist examined it and discovered PENICILLIN. This opened the door for the discovery of many marvelous anti-biotics. In an article entitled, "Anti-biotics That Come From Higher Plants", by P. S. Schaffer, et al, it is reported that 73 plant extracts were tested, seeking those with fungicidal properties. The most active were extracts obtained from Nasturtium, Jewelweed, wild Touch-me-not and Muskmelon. The ancient Indians did not know when they put some boiled-down juice of Jewelweed on an itchy spot that they were really treating a fungal disorder with 2-methoxy-1, 4-naptho-quinone, but that is what modern science isolated from the plants mentioned, a marvelous cure for athlete's foot, etc.!

The marvelous thing about plant medicines is that despite the Egyptians, Greeks, Assyrians, Chinese and early Hindus listing and identifying hundreds of types, the SURFACE HAS BEEN BARELY SCRATCHED! In the 1850's only 6,000 of the 350,000 plants that are known to exist today had been examined and classified. Some 4,000 species of plants that are "new" to the botanist today are added each year to the list! Of the 4,000 medicines now in use containing herbs, two-thirds have been developed in the last 10 years! Recently two native American plants with strong anti-tumor properties were discovered — the purple Meadow rue of Wisconsin and the Florida plant, Elephantopus elatus. A list was recently made of 1500 plants with reputed medicinal value growing in one state alone. Cancer researchers have found anti-cancer effects in nearly 3,000 diferent plants throughout the world!

The value of plant drugs is assessed in "Cancer Chemotherapy Report No. 7", issued by the Public Health Service: "To sum up, the empirical application of plants to the ailing human body over thousands of years has resulted in certain observed effects interpreted as beneficial, and has culminated in the development of many useful drugs for a number of diseases. If there is any hope in a chemical treatment for cancer, it is reasonable to believe that such an agent is as likely to originate from a plant as from pure synthesis." Consequently a "green boom" is sweeping over our land, with scientists and commercial drug producers discovering gold among the greens. They are sending out more than a thousand plant detectives every year to track down and investigate ancient herbal cures. A jungle researcher exploring the wilds of the Amazon may encounter a tribe using a certain plant to cure some type of insanity (as one did recently) and excitedly wire back to the U.S., "Investigate plant N° L57-67 as possible cure for schizophrenia." One researcher recently brought back 80 plants that had been traditionally used in just one East African tribe for medicines and said, "We're literally leaving no plant unturned." Schizophrenia afflicts millions in the world's modern cities today but a plant cure is reported being used in the jungles of the Amazon!

Before 1900 introduced the Age of Synthetic Drugs, 80% of all medicines in use were obtained from roots, stems and leaves of plants. Then a proud reaction set in and man turned to the test tube to make his own medicines artificially from various chemicals. But now a top researcher comments: "We've come full circle. Back in the 1800's, fully 80 per cent of the medicines were plant derived. Gradually, researchers turned more and more to chemicals, both organic and inorganic. Today, half the curatives in the average family's medicine cabinet are products of somebody's test tube. And only 30 per cent are plant based. Now, almost out of desperation, we're going back to nature— back to plants. For good as the test tube is, it hasn't cured man's great cripplers— arthritis, heart trouble, insanity, asthma and cancer." Drug companies are now gambling millions of dollars a year on the search for "green gold."

What happens when a report is heard of a new type of medicinal plants? Investigators are sent to secure samples of the plant and then it is shipped back to the laboratories for detailed analysis— it is put through the research wringer. Grinders reduce the plant's parts to tiny fragments; chemicals dissolve out its hundreds of separate substances; electrostatic machines isolate other substances; infrared spectrophotometers double-check the elements for purity. Finally there may remain, after years of study, some new or unknown chemical or crystal with possible curative powers. But Dr. Alfred Taylor of the University of Texas states, "We've never had as much success with chemicals invented by man as we're having with plant extracts." Since a scientist admits these facts, we might ask, "Why is this so?" Herbalists and naturopaths have a ready answer from nature. We know for instance, that plants and plants only can transmute inorganic elements into the organic substances which become the food of animals and man. Therefore when we use plants medicinally we are employing active organic substances which are in HARMONY with our own physical composition. Chemical drugs are inert materials often incompatible with the chemistry of our bodies — an added reason for the superiority of herbal medicines!

Take for example, the popular birth control Pill so widely spoken of in modern society; it was developed from a Mexican Camote plant used for this purpose by Mexican Indians. But science is impatient with collecting sufficient plants to make up Pills for the vast number using Pills, so science proceeds to artificially build a chemical compound SIMILAR to the active element in the plant. BUT this is then a synthetic or artificial hormone, isolated from the total complex of the natural plant itself (which perhaps had some built-in safeguards). So what happens? Now the Pill has dangerous side-effects which the TIME magazine of January 26, 1970, says includes reactions such as weight gains, forming of blood clots, causing of strokes, raising of blood pressure, migraine headaches, diabetes, liver disease, breast cancer and possibly rheumatoid arthritis as well as psychological changes! Charges exist that the Pill also damages genetic structure and may damage the unborn fetus, like thalidomide. But while it is being investigated, millions and millions continue to be sold and used and an estimated 250 women die each year from its effects! Or listen to this description of a commonly used drug from a doctor's handbook, warning about its side-effects — but does the doctor warn his patients? — "Triamcinoline is a steroid... capable of causing toxic (poisonous) effects ... also likely to cause flushing of the face, muscle cramps, sweating, mental depression, and a peculiar weakness of pelvic, trunk, and shoulder muscles." If we were to list here all the possible bad reactions of many modern super drugs, including the final penalty of DEATH exacted, you would begin to ask yourself, "IS NOT THE MEDICINE WORSE THAN THE DISEASE?" This is a good reason for the superiority of herbal medicines.

The American naturalist Thoreau wrote, "A man may esteem himself happy when that which is his food is also his medicine." Herbal doctors rely on small doses over a long period of time rather than on powerful doses all at once. The plant medicines, usually of low potency (highly diluted), are designed to first purify the bloodstream and restore normal functioning of the ductless glands. Purification, restoration, and gradualism help the body to rejuvenate itself with its natural defenses to the point of recuperation. Some medical doctors scoff at the diluted, low potency of homeopathic medicines but the low power of a NATURAL substance is infinitely better than the radical, high-powered artificial substance. How does the scientist know what subtle change chemical synthesis may have effected in turning an organic into an inorganic medicine? For example, one plant extract made only with water was discovered which had a remarkable effect on the agglutination of red blood cells —ONLY ONE PART OF THE PLANT FLUID TO 16,000 PARTS OF WATER WAS NECESSARY! Think of it! Can nature's packaging be improved upon in medicines?

This is the very finest point of herbal medicines — their greatest virtue is not only their curative powers but their preventive powers. Many flavorful and fragrant herbs and plants may be used as food and drink for the well rather than merely medicine for the sick. The regular use of certain plants and herbs not as medicine but as part of the daily diet has some prophylactic or preventive value in warding off illness. If we made more use of these fresh green herbs and plants, not as medicine, but as part of our daily diet, their high vitamin and mineral contents would build up our resistance to disease and help prevent us from becoming a nuisance to the already overworked doctors of modern society. Moreover, preventive medicine is not as expensive a proposition as curative medicine. It is better to have a safety fence at a dangerous mountain curve than an ambulance waiting down in the valley to pick up the pieces afterwards.

A few other examples of modern uses discovered for ancient herbal medicines are as follows. Curare, an arrow poison of the Amazonian jungle Indians, has been developed into sedatives and a whole line of antispasmodics useful in spastic paralysis and multiple sclerosis. Abbot Laboratories announced the discovery of a drug effective against hardening of the arteries — it was discovered in Safflower oil. A still unanalysed plant in Mexico was observed to have the power with only a few picked leaves to instantly stop any wound from bleeding when the leaves were placed on the cut. No drug known today comes close to duplicating this feat.

Much research recently done with seeds shows that such seeds as those of the Privet, Dog rose, White acacia, Common Ash and Honey locust contain powerful anti-biotic substances. Effective diuretics were found in the seeds of Caraway, Sweet Fennel, and Anise, which are all particularly safe and commonly used as spices and flavorings. Anti-cancer alkaloids have been discovered in the Periwinkle plant and have stimulated much more research for anti-cancer elements in plants.

Other outstanding examples of medicines from plants are Quinine for malaria from Cinchona bark; Chaulmoogra oil for leprosy from the seeds of the Chaulmoogra tree; aspirin is a much-used synthetic drug modelled after the natural salts of the Wintergreen plant; a powerful fungicide known as leptonin was developed from Bitterroot wood; country people have used the plant known as "Devil's shoestrings" to kill vermin for centuries — only in the last 20 years have chemists learned to use this same plant as rat poison under the name of Red Squill. Of 4,000 medicines now in use containing herbs, two-thirds have been developed in the last ten years. Often yesterday's worthless weed is tomorrow's valuable herb. A wild yam root (Camote) from Mexico has been discovered to be a vegetable hormone source of cortisone and the basis for the new birth control pills. Colchicum plants have provided colchicine, a specific for gout; Ipecac, the source of emetine, is used in the treatment of amoebic dysentery; even the deadly Nightshade plant has become the source of a useful sedative.

Because of medical and industrial demand, yearly $300 million worth of herbs are sold in the U. S. Thousands of tons of plants are now being used every year by the main pharmaceutical companies and the trade is growing by leaps and bounds. $25 million is being spent yearly in research into plant medicines. But one writer on this subject. (D. P. Mannix) notes: "Millions have been spent trying to produce the organic chemicals from medicinal plants synthetically. In almost every case it has been a long and expensive, and not always very successful effort. It took 134 years for chemists to learn how to synthesize morphine, and it was 58 years after tropine, an eye medicine, was first synthesized before the process could be made cheap enough for commercial purposes. The so-called 'synthetics', in turn, are often made by substituting other plants for the originals. The synthesizing of natural compounds, therefore, has increased the demand for herbs rather than diminished it. We still need these wild plants."

Plant medicines are having a tremendous revival today. In 1963, out of 300 million prescriptions written in the U. S. by medical doctors, 47% contained as their active principal ingredient (or one of the two most principal ingredients) a medicine of natural origin. We are steadily learning from science that man's medicine is exactly where the Bible has always said it was— in the plant kingdom. The writing of 39 books has been attributed to the wisest man, king Solomon. One of these was an herbal book supposedly giving the botanical remedies for every disease. Unfortunately this book was reported to have been destroyed in the Fall of Jerusalem in 70 A.D. The Bible is full of references to herbs (balm, myrtle, figs, coriander seed, camphire, spikenard, saffron, calamus, cinnamon, frankincense, myrrh, aloes, hyssop, etc.). We may well believe that there is not a single disease in man that may not have its remedy or cure in some herb or other, if we but knew which plant and where to find it. Of course the element of faith is also essential in all healing. The Roman writer Seneca said, "It is part of the cure to wish to be cured." And Christ said, "Thy faith hath made thee whole." Herbal medicines are no substitute for faith but can indicate a return to a simple Bible faith that what God has prescribed must be good.

For further study on the subject of this chapter, these books are helpful: "STALKING THE HEALTHFUL HERBS", by Euell Gibbons (David McKay Co., Inc., 1966, 303 pp.); "USING PLANTS FOR HEALING", by Nelson Coon (Hearthside Press, Inc., 1963, 272 pp.); "THE JUNGLE SEARCH FOR NATURE'S CURES", by Nicole Maxwell (Ace Books, Inc., 1961, 256 pp.); "GREEN MEDICINE", by Margaret B. Krieg (Rand McNally & Co., 1964, 453 pp.); "NATURE'S MEDICINES", by Richard Lucas (Award Books, N.Y., 1966, 251 pp.). Two helpful articles are: "In Search of Plants that Cure", by James Joseph (POPULAR MECHANICS Magazine, April, 1960) and "The Men Who Dig for Green Gold", by D. P. Mannix (TRUE Magazine, May, 1968).

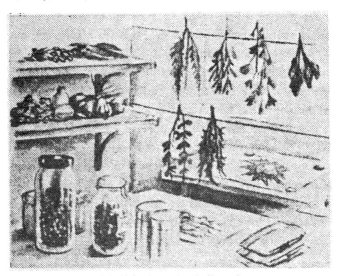

Medicinal Herbs Collected

Since I started studying and writing on the subject of medicinal plants, our whole family has gotten interested in the subject. My children report from time to time about the various plants they have discovered locally which have different healing actions. My two oldest girls were telling me the other day that they took sap from orange and lemon trees and boiled it until it became like taffy — it felt so good that they began putting it on cuts and wounds and it caused them to close up and stop bleeding. Another remedy they discovered on their own was to take the nectar from local honeysuckle and rub it on cuts and scratches — it takes away the pain and quickly heals them up. A neighbor told us the other day about a tree bark that is locally used to heal stomach ulcers; a man who had not been helped by numerous high-priced medications began taking a boiled infusion from the bark and soon his ulcers disappeared. (By the way, coffee causes the lining of the stomach to secrete large quantities of hydrochloric acid. Ulcer patients should not drink coffee). Another American friend down here in Costa Rica told us about a native plant called Saragondi — the leaves are used to make a tea which heals rheumatism. Many illnesses of modern civilized man are simple vitamin and mineral deficiencies. Calcium and Vitamin D deficiencies give rise to many headaches, muscle cramps and joint pains. As yet the richest source of these indispensable vitamins and minerals is scarcely being tapped — HERBS. Take for example, Parsley, which has been discovered to have 22,500 Vitamin A units per ounce, 1,050 Vitamin C units per ounce (while orange juice has only 300), and furthermore Parsley has 5.763 milligrams of iron per ounce! God has prescribed long ago a medicine that man cannot imitate with any artificial product — fresh, green, growing HERBS! The University of Costa Rica is doing research on medicinal herbs. One of the University professors of archaeology says that in pre-Colombian days (prior to 1492), Costa Rica was widely known among the Indian civilizations as the best herb depositary in the whole Western Hemisphere. This is because Costa Rica is a zone where the vegetation of both North and South America may be found.

CHAPTER VI: Common Herbal Remedies, Classified by How They Work:

We trust the foregoing has whetted your appetite to learn more about God-given herbal remedies for the healing of mankind. This present book can only be in the nature of a brief survey of the subject and yet it would not be complete without a section of actual herbal remedies. Many herbal books classify the common remedies according to the various diseases, others classify the recipes as to the method by which they affect the body (for example, fighting fever, or soothing rheumatism, or relieving constipation, or relaxing nervous tension, etc.). In this section we have chosen to classify the herbal remedies by the second approach. Nevertheless, in the final chapter, a brief index is given also classifying the various common ailments and listing the pages on which their appropriate remedies are discussed. May we again here remind the reader, as we have repeatedly done, that it is impossible for any merely human author to have the omniscience to PRESCRIBE SPECIFICALLY for the ailments of a reading audience. All we can do is discuss what many have found to be helpful throughout history. This book is not meant to replace doctors but only to provide an introduction to a much neglected natural therapy.

The common herbal remedies discussed in the chapter will immediately raise the practical question, 'Where can the reader procure the herbal ingredients mentioned?' In the final chapter a list of companies and pharmacies selling these herbs is given. The numerous books mentioned as references for further study are available at bookstores listed in the final chapter. Furthermore, a directory of licensed, medical doctors who have been trained in homeopathic therapy can be procured by writing to an address listed in the final chapter. Thus the reader who seriously wished to investigate this subject further is not left without resources and references.

In becoming acquainted with any school of medical therapy, the layman is often confused from the start by its incomprehensible technical jargon, amounting to almost a secret language in code. Herbalism and homeopathy necessarily use some technical words but their meaning is easily grasped. For the convenience of the reader new to this vocabulary, I am here giving a brief list of the main types of herbal remedies, classified by their action. The reader is advised to casually read through all these categories and then especially study whichever class especially speaks to his condition. This is a list given for the purpose of repeated re-study and reference so it is good to first familiarize yourself with the various types of herbal action and then go to study more in detail the categories discussed.

GLOSSARY OF TYPES OF HERBAL MEDICINES:

ALTERATIVES — herbal medicines conducive to gradually correcting a poor condition by tonic action (as on the blood).

ANTI-BIOTICS — organic herbal medicines working selectively against harmful micro-organisms and infections.

ANTIHELMINTICS — expelling or destroying worms.

ANTIPYRETICS — any medicine for checking and preventing fever.

ANTIRHEUMATICS — having an effect counteracting rheumatism, arthritic inflammations of the joints and gout.

ANTISCOURBUTICS — food or medicine preventing or curing scurvy.

ANTISPASMODICS — relieving spasms, contractions, muscular tensions, and some headaches.

ANTISEPTICS — preventing mortification and infection.

APERIENTS — opening, mild and gentle laxatives.

APHRODISIACS — medicines restoring virility.

AROMATICS — agreeable, spicy, restorative inhalants, volatile oils, flavors and vapors.

ASTRINGENTS — contracting the fibres or tissues, checking discharges.

BITTER TONICS — stimulating secretions, and appetite.

CALMATIVES — Calming, soothing effect.

CARMINATIVES — have a pungent, warming effect on the stomach, expelling wind and gas, relieving colic and flatulence.

CATHARTICS — purges and laxatives.

CHOLAGOGUES — increasing the flow of bile, stimulating the cleansing of the liver and gall bladder.

COUNTERIRRITANTS — causing irritation or mild pain on the body's surface in order to relieve a deeper, more acute pain.

DEMULCENTS — softening effect, sheathing or lubricating internally.

DIAPHORETICS — producing perspiration.

DEOBSTRUENTS — clearing obstruction from the natural ducts of the body.

DIURETICS — increasing the secretion and flow of urine.

EMETICS — causing vomiting, as purge or antidote to poison.

EMOLLIENTS — softening, causing warmth, moisture, lotions for the skin.

EXPECTORANTS — stimulating saliva and spitting, the expulsion of mucous secretions and phlegm.

FEBRIFUGES — dispelling fever or allaying fever heat.

FUNGICIDALS — tending to kill fungal infections.

LAXATIVES — stimulating mild evacuation of the intestines and bowels.

NERVINES — strengthening the nerves, calming excitement.

NARCOTICS — powerful and dangerous drugs bringing a feeling of euphoria by depressing certain nerve centers.

PECTORALS — useful in diseases of the lung and chest.

POULTICE — a soft mass of crushed plant matter applied to the surface of the body.

PURGATIVES — promoting abundant and frequent evacuations of the bowels.

REFRIGERANTS — cooling effect, lowering body heat.

RUBEFACIENTS — reddening the surface of the skin or lining of a hollow organ by attracting the blood to that area.

SEDATIVES — depressing, calming, tranquilizing the vital powers.

SOPORIFICS — inducing sleep.

STIMULATIVES — exciting the vital power and nerves.

STOMACHICS — tonics stimulating and strengthening the stomach and appetite.

STYPTICS — checking or stopping bleeding.

SUDORIFICS — producing abundant perspiration or sweating.

THORACIC — herbs used to treat complaints of the lungs and bronchial tubes.

TRANQUILIZERS — having a calming effect.

VERMIFUGES — destroying worms.

VULNERARIES — washes, sprays, douches, used in swabbing, nasal sprays, etc.

If you are interested in knowing more about the properties of the herbs which shall be discussed in this chapter, the following books will be found to be very helpful. For those who would like details on how to collect and prepare their own herbs: "STALKING THE HEALTHFUL HERBS", By Euell Gibbons (David McKay., Inc., N.Y., 1966, 303 pp.); and, "USING PLANTS FOR HEALING", by Nelson Coon (Hearthside Press, Inc., 1963, 271 pp.). Lists of medicinal herbs and their properties can be found in: "THE HERBALIST", by Joseph E. Meyer, 1960, 304 pp.: "ABOUT HERBS", by Dr. Benedict Lust, 1961, 72 pp.; "CULPEPPER'S COMPLETE HERBAL", publ. by W. Foulsham Co., London, 430 pp.; "HERBAL MANUAL", by Harold Ward, L. N. Fouler & Co., London, 1967, 136 pp.; "THE SIMMONITE-CULPEPPER HERBAL REMEDIES", W. Foulsham & Co., London, 1957, 123 pp.; "PROVEN REMEDIES", by J. H. Oliver, Thorsons Publishers, Ltd., London, 1968, 92 pp.; "THE MODERN BOTANIC PRESCRIBER", by Aric F. Powell, L. N. Fowler Co., London, 1965, 136 pp.; "NATURE'S MEDICINES", by Richard Lucas, Award Books, N. Y., 1956, 251 pp. These and many more good books on this subject may be ordered from various book dealers listed in the final chapter.

It is well to add here again that the remedies we shall discuss in this chapter are in the nature of recipes commonly used for home consumption and first aid in the family and are not intended as technical prescriptions. Everyone has in their medicine chest some common home remedies. These herbal recipes were often used by our ancestors. If you cannot collect them personally from wayside or garden, most can be purchased from some herb company or homeopathic pharmacy (addresses in the final chapter). In the discussion of the various herbal remedies, you will notice that oftentimes more than a half-dozen herbs are listed together which have a certain effect (such as a tonic). The purpose of listing more than one is so that the person interested may make a tea compounded of several herbs with similar action and thus strengthen the working of the remedy. Most of these herbal ingredients can be purchased inexpensively for 50 cts. for a small box of any one herb, cleaned and cut and dried. It is about as much (or more) fun as cooking to prepare your own herbal teas, salves, etc. John Gerard said in 1597: "Nothing can be concocted, either delicate for the taste, dainty for smell, pleasant for sight, wholesome for the body, conservative for health, but it borroweth the relish of an herb, the juice of a plant, or the decoction of a root."

Remember that if your illness or discomfort does not respond readily to some simple home remedy, proceed as you would ordinarily and consult your doctor immediately. While it is true that it is your constitu tional right to prescribe for yourself, it is your own responsibility and the writers of herb books, sellers of herbs, etc, cannot guarantee any cures. Only God can cure through nature (or supernaturally); there is always a possibility that what has helped thousands of people over the course of the centuries may fail to help another individual. Remember too that you can spoil or cancel the effects of many or most herbal and homeopathic medicines by indulging in coffee, tobacco, alcoholic beverages, and even excessive use of salt.

HERBAL REMEDIES CLASSIFIED

ALTERATIVES: These are herbal medicines that aim at gradually correcting a poor condition by tonic action on the blood, etc. American Spikenard root (½ ounce simmered in 1½ pints of water) has been considerably used in rheumatic and general uric acid disorders as well as various skin diseases. As in most all herbal decoctions, the water is first heated and then removed when vigorously boiling, then the herb is put in and steeped for 15 minutes (with a saucer inverted over the cup to conserve the oils), before straining and drinking. Other helpful alteratives include Yellow Dock, Red Clover, Burdock Root, Dandelion Root, American Sarsaparilla, Sassafrass bark, Goldenseal root, Elderberry flower, etc. Homeopathic Sulphur 6X is a good blood purifier. Often eating foods rich in iron (potatoes in their skins, watercress, raw dandelion leaves) builds up the blood. Biochemical Ferrum phos. 3X or any good organic iron tonic is helpful in purifying and building up the blood. Garlic is a known blood cleanser. You will get much more benefit in general from fresh picked or dried herbs full of vitamins and minerals than from any synthetic supplement on the market. Happy is the man whose food is his medicine; the best medicinal foods are from wild herbs as processed foods often have lost much of their vitamin contents after being "shot through guns", colored, preserved and packaged.

ANTI-BIOTICS: Organic herbal medicines working selectively against harmful micro-organisms and infections. The commonest herbal anti-biotic and one of the most powerful that exists is garlic. It can be taken by eating the raw cloves of garlic, or taking ten drops of garlic oil three times daily, or by using garlic poultices, etc. Some health food companies have prepared excellent garlic oil capsules or garlic-parsley tablets made of dehydrated fresh garlic and parsley and the advantage of these is that you don't have as much sharp taste and smell. In 1944 an extract of the vital principle of garlic oil was made, called Allicin. Even in dilutions of 1 to 85,000 and 1 to 125,000, allicin showed up as a powerful bactericide, fighter of virus and infection. It has been used successfully in many countries in the treatment of such difficult diseases as typhoid fever, staphylococcus and streptococcus, amebic and bacillic dysentery, ptomaine poisoning, gangrene and even polio. It is not yet known exactly what makes garlic so powerful but it is suspected that besides the bactericidal and viricidal effects of the garlic oil, it contains unknown vitamins and hormones that work best in their natural state as part of the organic plant bulb. The odor of the garlic bulb is very diffusible and even when it is applied by rubbing or poultice to the soles of the feet, its odor will later be detected exhaled by the lungs!

Garlic has been widely used in treating tuberculosis and other diseases of the chest. It is also an expectorant, rubifacient, diuretic, stimulant, carminative, and aromatic. Because of its wide use in Russia for numerous infections and diseases, it has been called "Russian penicillin". It was used extensively in Bible times as well. It is known to have a strengthening and slightly laxative effect, disinfecting the contents of the stomach and intestines, fighting diarrhea, dyspepsia, sore throats, flu, etc. A German medical study in 1950 indicated that garlic oil is composed of various organic sulfides and disulfides which united with virus matter in such a way as to block and kill them yet without harming any beneficial body organism. Research is now going on with garlic injections in cancerous mice in which it has blocked and killed some types of malignancy. A Japanese scientist recently discovered that certain substances in garlic increase the body's capacity to assimilate vitamin B-1. It used to be said, "An apple a day keeps the doctor away"; if you are not afraid of the odor keeping EVERYBODY away, try a regular daily use of garlic to fortify your system against viral infections.

Since onions are a member of the same plant family as garlic (which is that part of the Lily family known as genus Allium, and includes chives and leek as well), it is interesting to know that fresh onion and onion juice have similar anti-biotic properties, though not as powerful as garlic. Many plants' essential oils seem to contain antibiotic effects, as yet imperfectly understood (see Aromatics). Before ridiculing plants as a source of anti-biotics, it is well to remember that penicillin was extracted from bread-mold (used for centuries by the Greeks to cure wounds) Anti-biotic substances have recently been discovered in the seeds of the Privet, Dog rose, White acacia, Common ash and Honey locust. It remains to be seen what marvellous substances will be discovered in the future in other seeds and nut-meats. Furthermore, an herbal anti-biotic like garlic does not have the bad side-effects of such synthetic anti-biotics as penicillin and others (allergic reactions, antibiotic super-infection, etc.)

ANTIHELMINTICS: These are herbs that expel or destroy worms. It is ironic that man rides in rockets to the moon while millions of men on earth still itch and squirm from worms and other parasites taking a free ride inside of man! Garlic kills round-worms and thread-worms and can thus also be classified as an antihelmintic. Others are Wormwood, Male Fern root, Elm bark, Flax seed, Jerusalem oak, Pumpkin seed, Pomegranate rind, Spigelia root. As some of these have powerful effects, it is best to consult your doctor or naturopathic practitioner on the proper dosages. If coconut husks are available, some ground to a powder and administered to a child after fasting will prove beneficial. Kamla and also Tansy flowers are effective (but strong); Chemopodium has a 91 per cent efficiency against hook-worm as compared with Thymol's 83%. But by all means consult your physician.

ANTIPYRETICS: These are any herbal medicines for checking and preventing fever. Oil of Sweet Birch, whose main active principle is Methyl Salicylate, is an antipyretic as well as an antirheumatic (rheumatism acts like a kind of "fever" in the joints). This oil is practically indistinguishable from oil of Wintergreen and again the active ingredient is salicylic acid, the major ingredient of aspirin. But how much better it is to use that which comes from the natural herb than the synthetic product! In the same category of herbs we find FEBRIFUGES, which have an effect of dispelling or allaying fevers. These include Witch-grass (1 ounce of dried roots to a pint of boiling water, drink a small glass three times daily); Aspen, Balsam Poplar, Calamus root, Common Balm, and Golden Seal are others in this class. Capsicum (Cayenne Pepper) brewed into tea or in powdered form in capsules (10 to 15 grains) is also taken internally for fevers. It has tremendous antiseptic and vitamin C properties. Most parents of young children realize that persistent high fevers can be dangerous and even lead to convulsions and brain damage. A persistent high-fever is immediate grounds for calling a doctor. Until he arrives, first- aid can be administered by cool, wet cloths bathing the forehead. Beware of much use of aspirin and bufferin as they can cause harmful side-effects (as well as being a potential source of death should children eat large quantities, thinking them to be candy).

ANTIRHEUMATICS: Herbal medicines having an effect counteracting rheumatism, arthritis, gout and etc. These are usually all disorders which require time to conquer as they may be the result of a long-poisoned system and require sensible dieting, fasting, bathing as well as internal and external medication. Baths with Epsom salts or with oil of Eucalyptus are helpful; oil of Wintergreen liniments and massaging the joints are helpful to many. A powerful homeopathic remedy is Rhus toxicodendron 30X, Rhododendron 30X, and Bryonia 30X, 10 drops of each daily, in a little water. This is what cured the present author after fasting, raw juices and vapor baths cleaned out my system. It is ironic that Rhus tox (poison ivy) is such a powerful agent for good in this disease but this is just another demonstration of homeopathy's "like cures like" rule. A highly diluted oil of Rhus tox is taken internally and seems to act as a swift counter-attack on the rheumatic joints. In bad cases, some use Rhus tox 10M (more potent). The systemic nature of these diseases must be recognized so that therapy can be directed to the whole system and not just the affected joints. If this is not done, the joints will eventually deteriorate. The cure must be accomplished by the healing power inherent in the body itself — it must be allowed to overthrow the poisons shackling it and through systemic renovation recuperate. To cut down on uric acid in the system, sugar, fat meats and white flour should be curtailed. Some also find relief from trying homeopathic bee-sting tablets, as the formic acid seems to relieve rheumatic inflammation. A strong tea made by pouring a cup of boiling water over a teaspoonful of chopped Arbovitae foliage, letting it steep for ten minutes, is found helpful by many. See Aromatics for more on Rheumatism and Diuretics for more on Gout. Many doctors also believe there is a definite Vitamin C deficiency present in all rheumatic cases and have found massive doses of Vitamin C to stimulate recuperation from rheumatism and arthritis; eating of plentiful citrus fruits is very helpful — especially oranges and drinking much juice from limes.

ANTISCORBUTICS: herbal medicines (or fruits and vegetables) preventing or curing scurvy. Any plant that contains significant amounts of Vitamin C, and most plants do, is an antiscorbutic. Juice of the citrus fruits is especially good to counteract scurvy (British sailors came to be called "Limeys" because their ships required daily drinking of lime juice against scurvy). Less palatable but even more powerful in Vitamin C is Pine Needle tea, made by pouring 1 pint of boiling water over 1 ounce of fresh White Pine needles chopped fine (add a squeeze of lemon and some honey to improve the taste). Richer yet in Vitamin C is Rose Hip tea; a single cup of pared rose hips may contain as much Vitamin C as 10 to 12 DOZEN oranges and of course one cup of rose hips will make many cups of tea. Also used are dandelion roots and sarsaparilla. The Vitamin C content of garlic and of cayenne pepper is very high.

ANTISPASMODICS: herbs relieving spasms, contractions, muscular tensions and some types of headaches. These include Scullcap, Catnip, Spearmint, Chamomile, Hop Flowers, Purslane, etc. Oil of Peppermint has a very strong antispasmodic action, making it valuable for sudden pains and stomach cramps. Mint has been known as a remedy since the time of the ancient Egyptians. References to it in the Bible as a tithing contribution indicate it was a medium of exchange, greatly valued. It was also used by the ancients to scent the bath, as a restorative, and a flavoring in foods and for more disagreeably tasting medicines. Tea made from Red Raspberry leaves is widely used to relieve the severity and length of labor pains and facilitate delivery. Expectant mothers drinking

Red Raspberry leaf tea every morning during pregnancy are helped to have easy labor. The leaves contain some unknown factor helping prevent miscarriage in addition to easing of cramps. The tea is made by steeping an ounce of dried leaves in 20 ounces of boiling water. Drink 10 to 20 ounces of tea daily, sweetened with honey. We have experienced the benefits of this in our own family. Migraine headaches are treated with such homeopathic remedies as kali carb., six tablets every half hour during an attack, and every eight hours during intervals; Arnica too is very good. Many severe headaches can be relieved by taking a deep, hot foot bath for five to ten minutes, with or without added mustard (while bathing the feet apply a folded handkerchief to the forehead, well-dampened with equal parts of cold water and vinegar and renew frequently). Oil of rosemary applied to the temples and rubbed in is good.

ANTISEPTICS: are herbal medicines preventing mortification and infection. The ancients used to use wine to wash wounds (alcohol sterilizing most germs) or even bathe them with tears (human tears contain powerful germicidal properties, believe it or not). In the South Pacific, quantities of sea-weed were used and their rich iodine content sterilized the wounds. Sphagnum moss has been discovered to have powerful antiseptic and antibiotic qualities. Sassafrass, Boneset, Wormwood and Persimmon bark have been recorded as having antiseptic qualities. Elecampane (Scabwort) is both an antiseptic and bactericide. Juice of the onion is a powerful antiseptic and in case of a bee or wasp sting, a freshly cut onion poultice held over the sting or bite will hinder infection, draw out the poison and anesthetize or remove the pain. We have used this numerous times in our family so that when the onion is applied at once, the bite or sting does not swell up but dwindles away. Furthermore, oil of citronella acts as an insect repellent to gnats and mosquitoes (rub it on your wrists, neck and ankles when going for a hike in the woods). Pennyroyal oil applied to horse harness and dog collars acts as a repellent to fleas. The black Maltese fungus was famous for centuries to heal wounds.

Garlic has a very powerful antiseptic action. One doctor specialising in treatment of tuberculosis tried 56 different treatments and concluded: "Garlic is the best individual treatment found to get rid of germs." The Chinese have long recognized the valuable antiseptic properties of garlic. In Brazil, Garlic was discovered to have effected 100 per cent cures of 300 patients with intestinal infections ranging from enterocolitis to amebic dysentery. Not only in pulmonary infections, intestinal infections, but also in skin infections and wounds garlic has been found a powerful bactericide. During World War II, thousands of tons of garlic were purchased by the British government for treating the wounds of soldiers and not one so treated developed blood poisoning or gangrene. Pimples disappear without leaving scars if rubbed several times daily with garlic (although it must be remembered that purification of the skin and prevention of pimples must take place through the blood). Experiments carried out in Russia in 1945 proved that introducing colonies of bacteria into garlic juice caused them to completely cease all movement within three minutes. Conversely, when garlic juice was added to large colonies of bacteria, the bacteria moved immediately to the edges of the container, trying to escape, and within ten minutes all were dead. Dilution of the garlic juice reduces its efficiency and the freshly prepared juice is more effective than that preserved for several months. An old Spanish-American cure for amebas is to grind up from 8 to 15 cloves of garlic and drink with a half liter of warm milk (using the mixture also as an enema is another alternative); then for prevention of recurrence, always eat raw garlic and onions mixed with the rest of your food. After living in the tropics in an area heavily infested with amebas and having constant trouble off and on with them for eight months, and having tried at least eight or nine different synthetic drugs supposed to kill amebas, I was not cured of them until I began to regularly eat garlic with every meal. Since doing that, I have not had a single problem with amebas! Considering how inexpensive and harmless garlic is, it annoys me to think of how much money I wasted on dangerous drugs uselessly. A Garlic clove inserted in the ear relieves many earaches.

The ancients discovered by trial and error in hot or tropical climates that if meats were cooked in certain spices, they would not putrefy for days (and if cooked in Mustard oil, some foods not for weeks). Thus spices were used as powerful germicides to preserve foods and arrest spoilage. They learned to bring combinations of spices together to form the basis for the various curries, to render the foods not only more tasty but safer from spoilage and food poisoning. Cinnamon is a very powerful germicide; the scientist Cavel took beef broth infected with sewage-tank water, added to one sample Cinnamon oil diluted to 4 parts in 1000, to another sample oil of Cloves diluted to 2 parts in 1000, and the germs in both samples were completely destroyed! When carbolic acid was used, the strength of the solution had to be increased to 5 or 6 parts in 1000, yet how many people realize that Clove and Cinnamon oils are more powerful antiseptics than carbolic acid? Other spices such as Cumin, Caraway, Fennel, Cinnamon, Nutmeg, Cloves, Pepper, Turmeric and red Chilis preserve fats and prevent them from turning rancid and decaying. Other herbs are added with certain foods to counteract their bad effects: Fennel with all fish, Mint with pea soup (against flatulence), Savory with beans, Sweet marjoram with pork, goose and other fat meats. The best doctor is the cook. A meal of any kind without the benefit of spices for health and taste is like a house without windows! Flavoring herbs are generally added to foods shortly before they are finished cooking — otherwise the heat dissipates their action.

APERIENTS: Mild and gentle herbal laxatives; these include teas made of Witch-grass, Burdock, Fringe-tree, Chicory, Blue Flag, Elderberry, Dandelion, and Violets. Many of these already made-up in teabags can be purchased at your local health food store or ordered from some herb house. Nothing poisons the whole system like toxic wastes accumulating in that veritable sewer, the human digestive tract. Keep it clean and active!

APHRODISIACS: herbal medicines restoring sexual virility. It is best to consult your naturopathic practitioner or doctor on this area, as only a doctor can adequately diagnose this condition and prescribe a suitable remedy. This is a moral area in which much mischief could be done by unwise public discussion. There also exist herbal ABORTEFA-CIENTS to cause abortion, but we who believe life is sacred would not want to discuss such things publicly and thereby give cause for possible mischief, or even murder. Most states have very strict laws against abortion and only in the case of life or death for the mother would doctors prescribe abortion. It is. well known that the modern birth-control pills are based on herbal extracts from a Mexican plant but the result of wide use of such things has been an upswing in immorality and further downgrading of the sacredness of marriage. In the ancient world there was much abuse of aphrodisiacs, abortefacients and indiscriminate birth control; the result was a carnival of lust, the debasement of morality, the decline of religion and the family, and the collapse of civilization into degeneracy. This decline and fall was invariably followed by barbarism. Powerful herbal NARCOTICS also exist but woe to the amateur who meddles with such things leading to death and addiction. God gave herbs to heal, not to kill and enslave mankind.

AROMATICS: agreeable, spicy, restorative inhalants, volatile oils, flavors and vapors. We are today in naturopathy on the verge of discovery and exploration of a whole new area of herbal therapy using volatile oils extracted from plants. Little is known yet technically of how the body diffuses these volatile plant oils throughout the entire system so thoroughly and quickly but that it does so cannot be doubted. We have already mentioned how garlic rubbed on the soles of the feet can later be detected on the breath! Since the feet are vital areas of nerve endings leading to all parts of the body, is the vital oil transmitted by the nervous system? It is known in the psychology of smell that strong, volatile odors can be inhaled and quickly diffused throughout the body, causing marked mental and physical effects. How is it done? Through the nose into the lungs and then into the blood stream? Whatever the mechanism, the body readily distributes strong odors carrying tiny particles of volatile oils. Also volatile plant oils ingested in the stomach are quickly distributed throughout the body. Is it osmosis? It is again the blood stream? The whole therapy is only in its infancy as yet and it is strongly suspected that some volatile plant oils are powerful enough not only to pass into the body cells but even to disarrange cellular structure; it does not behoove anyone to experiment lightly with this.

However, over the centuries of human history, trial and error have demonstrated beneficial, therapeutic effects from some oils and harmful effects from others. We are here concerned only with mentioning common, beneficial plant essences or oils which can be classed among the herbalist's home remedies. Many of these are from common spices and flavorings and it is now understood that their ancient function of preventing deterioration and corruption in foods has a parallel in their antiseptic and germicidal qualities. Spices were used originally not because of their good flavor but because of their food preservative qualities. In these days of frightful, artificial food additives which can preserve foods by rendering them poisonous, we must not lightly assume that all that preserves is necessarily bad. Capsicum or Cayenne Red Pepper is used freely throughout the tropics as an herb to eat, chew on, and brew up into tea in order to disinfect the body, fight colds, fever and flu, and build up resistance to contagious diseases. The type of oils which seem most effective in Pneumotherapy (or Pneumatotherapy — the inhaling of herbal oils as vapor) are the volatile oils rather than the glyceride oils. Volatile oils are distilled, essential oils capable of passing off readily into vapor form. This likely accounts for their easy diffusibility throughout the body (whether by skin, lungs, blood, stomach, nerves or tissues).

Aromatics refer to the odors arising from a substance, its perfume, fragrance, exhalation, suspiration. It refers to the essential quality or spirit of the oil rising. Perhaps this is one reason why God chose to use oil as a symbol of the Holy Spirit and why anointing with oil was a commonly practised Bible ordinance in sanctifying, consecrating and healing. A subtle vapor pervading all the being would easily remind us of the action of the Holy Spirit infilling our lives with His love and holiness. So aromatic oils easily diffuse themselves throughout the body. Aromatic herbs include Anise seed, Fennel seed, Cloves, Catnip, Sassafras, Caraway, Sweet Flag, Wild Ginger, Peppermint, Tansy, Spearmint, Lovage, Black Pepper, Cinnamon, Camphor, Cayenne Pepper, Horseradish, Hyssop, Nutmeg, Pennyroyal, Sarsaparilla, White Pepper, Wintergreen etc. Most have a stimulant action, in addition to their other qualities. Who has not heard of using spirits of ammonia as a restorative inhalant for those fainting? Herbal aromatics are similar in action but less harsh and more beneficial to the whole system. Many essential oils of flowers have yet to be investigated for their therapeutic values and effects on the body. Ancient Greeks and Romans used incense for its medicinal values as well as religion. Pliny gives long lists of scents and perfumes as remedies for many diseases. The word "perfume" itself means *per* (by) *fume* (smoke). Frankincense, myrrh, rose, violet, iris, lily and other perfume-incenses were used in curative therapies — the patient inhaling the vapor from the burning or steaming perfumes. Who has not heard how some asthmatics get relief from inhaling medicated herbal smoke or fumes?

Hugo Hertwig, in his outstanding volume entitled "KNAURS HEILPFLANZENBUCH", has a very good discussion (pp. 240-244) on the therapeutic action of the ethereal or volatile oils of various herbs. They are actually found in all parts of the plants and one wonders if they might not be the main curative agent in all herbal and homeopathic medicines, the vital spirit of each plant, as it were. Ethereal or volatile oils have demonstrated strong anti-biotic characteristics. Naturally, in their working they show pronounced differences. They have been variously introduced to the body: inhaling, rubbing into the skin (which is more permeable for plant-stuffs than one would think), bath supplements, ingestion by mouth, and injection. Hertwig believes that the oils penetrate into the body and work on the central nervous system. By way of the lungs the vapors are taken on and absorbed by the whole body. The volatile oils are amazingly pervasive. Anyone who has ever taken even a small quantity of oil of turpentine, for example, can recognize the odor of violets in the urine afterwards! Garlic oil compresses applied to the feet cause the breath to smell of garlic! Truly man is fearfully and wonderfully made — not just a collection of different parts but a harmonious whole closely bound together in the golden network of nerves, blood vessels and interlocking cells. It is exactly in the action of volatile oils on the body system that again the homeopathic principle of diluted potencies is proven rational. To introduce too great a crowd of volatile oils into the system might conceivably damage the cells and the protoplasmic structure. Massive dosage could be extremely dangerous as a little goes a long way!

Rubbed outwardly, many volatile oils have a rubefacient effect on the skin, reddening it and dilating the blood vessels. Taken inwardly, in the form of herbal teas, they have a mild, stimulating effect on the appetite, stimulate peristalsis and the secretion of saliva, quicken the heartbeat and perfume the breath. Volatile oils are purchasable in the local pharmacies; often they are mixed in with prescription medicines so as to give a pleasing taste and odor to otherwise bitter medicines. What is not clearly understood is that they may also act as a vehicle carrying the other medicines more readily throughout the body! To mention just a few of the valuable, volatile oils, these have an antiseptic, stimulating and germicidal effect: Pine oil (purified), Thyme oil, Camomile oil, Eucalyptus oil, Oil of Peppermint, Oil of Horseradish, Fennel oil, Juniper oil, Parsley oil, Oil of Sage, and Wormwood oil. For antirheumatic effect, the following are useful: Oil of Birch bark, Oil of Wintergreen, Oil of Calamus, Mustard Oil, Camphor Oil. These should be applied externally by massage.

For inhalation for the lungs and respiratory system, it is best to have professional advice and prescription but these are the ones commonly used: Oil of Dwarf Pine, Oil of Spruce, Eucalyptus oil, Thyme oil. For severe whooping cough, Oil of Cypress and Thyme oil are used. Various kinds of vaporizers may be used or even atomizers for throat and nasal spray. It should be remembered that tiny quantities only should be used. Who has not seen a sick child with a bad chest cold greatly helped by vaporizing in the sick room some volatile oil or medicine? If you examine the ingredients of some common "vapor rubs" you will find one contains menthol (mint oil extract), camphor, oil of Eucalyptus, Nutmeg oil, oil of cedar, turpentine, Thyme oil. Another frequent addition to such preparations is Oil of Wintergreen. A popular commercial inhaler contains menthol, camphor, oil of Wintergreen, oil of Sassafrass, Ephedrine (from the Ephedra plants), etc., all serving together as a decongestant. A steam bath of Shave Grass may also relieve kidney and bladder troubles.

Other volatile aromatic herb oils include refined Turpentine oil with a depressant effect on the nervous system while the oils of Chamomile, Valerian and Angelica seed (Archangelica officinalis) have a calmative or sedative effect. Oil of Capsicum (Cayenne Red Pepper) is a powerfully volatile stimulant. The Cayenne Pepper itself is one of the most wonderful herb medicines which we have. It makes a good poultice for rheumatism, pleurisy, sores and wounds. Taken internally, it is a stimulant, antispasmodic, sudorific and laxative.

By far the most versatile and far-reaching of all the volatile oils is Garlic oil. We have already mentioned numerous times the various effects of Garlic such as bactericidal, antibiotic, antiseptic, viricidal, stimulant, expectorant, diuretic, rubefacient, antihelmintic, nervine, carminative, etc. Garlic is used as an ointment, in compresses, poultices, as internal medicine taken by mouth (raw juice, drops in solution, chewing the bulbs, or swallowing cloves of the Garlic, Garlic perles or tablets). Raw garlic juice is inhaled in whooping cough and pulmonary tuberculosis. The oil in which Garlic has been fried is a useful liniment for rheumatic pains. But Russian clinics and hospitals use Garlic almost entirely in the form of volatile extracts. These are not taken by mouth but are vaporized and inhaled. Garlic is truly a Healing Bulb with wide effects. No wonder the Pharaohs of Egypt were always careful to provide their workers and slaves with onions, leek and Garlic — to maintain a high level of healthy efficiency and a low level of illness absenteeism. It has been estimated that the equivalent of $2 million was spent by Pharaoh Cheops, during the construction of his pyramid, on maintaining the supply of Garlic for his work gangs! Long live Garlic (—and the man who eats it)! A modern-day revival of the ancient therapies of inhaling and rubbing in volatile plant oils is a step in the right direction health-wise. Try it and be surprised at the results

ASTRINGENTS: herbal medicines that contract the fibres or tissues, checking discharges. They are used as external washes, lotions, gargles, mouthwashes, etc. Just a few of the many are: Agrimony, Alum, Bayberry, Black Cherries, Black willow bark, Kola nuts, Logwood, Sage herb, Uva Ursi leaves, Witch Hazel twigs, Blackberry root, etc. All of these can be procured in powdered or other form at any herbal company and mixed into liquid washes. They may be made stronger by longer boiling or steeping. Why not experiment on making your own mouthwash and save a lot of money wasted on commercial products? Alum put on canker sores in the mouth soon dries them up; also Golden Seal powder has the same effect. The ancient Greek 'father of medicine', Hippocrates, recommended cleaning the teeth with a ball of wool that had been dipped in honey and them rinsing the mouth out with a mixture of dill, aniseed, myrrh and white wine (note the volatile oils added to an alcohol base). One old-fashioned but effective dentifrice or "tooth power" is simply mixing salt and bicarbonate of soda in equal parts. An excellent mouthwash can be made at home by adding rose water to plain water — experiment to see how many drops of the rose water you need. It leaves the mouth feeling pleasantly tingling and fragrant. Most sore throats will yield to sucking garlic cloves and letting the juice trickle down into the throat. Sassafrass bark infused in Rose Water makes a soothing and refreshing eye lotion. Capsicum (Red Pepper) in solution makes a good antiseptic mouth wash and gargle for sore throats.

Pleasantly astringent bath salts can be made by mixing three or four drams of oil of rose, oil of lavender, oil of jasmine, or whatever is your favorite, with 14 ounces of bicarbonate of soda and two ounces of potassium carbonate. Put a tablespoonful in the bath. Another pleasant, effervescent bath salts can be made up by crushing and mixing well together 5 ounces of tartaric acid, 5 ounces of bicarbonate of soda, and 3 ounces of corn-starch; for scent, add a few drops of rose geranium oil, oil of rosemary or oil of lavender. Put bath salts into the hot water just before getting in.

One well-known astringent herb tonic for the skin was known as "Hungary Water" and compounded of 12 ounces of rosemary, 1 ounce of lemon peel, 1 ounce of orange peel, 1 ounce of mint, 1 ounce of balm, 1 pint of rose water, 1 pint of alcohol, mixed together and let stand for several weeks to blend. Then the liquid was rubbed into the skin after bathing. Another herb tonic for the skin includes 1 ounce mint, 1 ounce sage, 1 ounce rosemary, 1 ounce lavender, 1 ounce mixed spices, 1 ounce camphor, 1 quart of white vinegar, 1 pint of alcohol, 2 ounces of myrrh, 2 ounces of benzoin. The resultant mixture can be rubbed on the skin or added in small amounts to bath water. Aromatic, fragrant, pungent herbs remain nature's best cleansers and rejuvenators of the skin, while commercial cosmetics are often full of harmful chemical additives derived from coal tar and commercial soaps full of harsh chemicals and fats.

BITTER TONICS: These are herbals stimulating secretions and appetite. Many a drug store or supermarket nowadays can sell you a bottle of "bitters" for your appetite, made up of common herbs. The commonest herbal ingredients are Angostura bark, Barberry root, Bayberry leaves, Bogbean herb, Chamomile flowers, Dandelion root, Gentian root, Hops flowers, Mugwort herb, Quassia chips, Serpentaria root, Wild Cherry bark, Wormwood herb, Yellow Root, etc. All of these are available from most herbal companies. Usually a teaspoonful or two of one herb is poured upon a pint of boiling water and a small glass drunk every morning before breakfast. Already blended mixtures of these "bitters" can be purchased ready-made for those who do not relish the work of collecting or selecting and mixing their own. But remember that the best spur to appetite is hard work and avoidance of overindulgence in food and drink. He who gets up from the table a little bit hungry rather than overstuffed will not be laid down so quick in the grave.

CALMATIVES: are botanicals with a calming, soothing effect. In an age of tension and anxiety when millions are practically addicted to strong chemical tranquilizers that have injurious side-effects damaging to the liver, it is good to consider returning to simple, herbal tranquilizers. Most common are the following, generally taken as a warm tea with honey upon retiring (honey itself has a pronounced calmative effect — try a spoonful on screaming children wakened by nightmares): Catnip herb, Chamomile flowers, Fennel seed, Hops, Linden flowers. Often your local health food store or drug store can supply you with a simple blend of calmative herbs, not needing a prescription; one type is called CALM-ETS and contains Orange Flowers, Valerian, Passion Flower, Celery Seed, Catnip and Hops. Another is called BIRAL and contains Corydalis cavo, Centranthus ruber, Valerian, Avena sativa, and Passion Flower. These herbal tranquilizers tend to lessen the sensitivity and excitability of the central nervous system without impairing the powers of concentration. Most synthetic sedatives (such as phenobarbital) are, if not actually addicting, accompanied by undesirable side-effects such as dizziness, depression and tiredness. These herbals in general are non-habit forming. Remember too, there is no substitute for peace and contentment coming from confession and forgiveness of sins and trust in God through Christ even in this tense, modern age. Millions are "doped up" who need to be spiritually "cleaned up".

A little known fact about one of the major causes of stress and tension in modern civilization is that NOISE can cause physiological changes. Former Surgeon General William H. Stewart reported: "It has been demonstrated that noise can cause physiological changes. These include cardiovascular, glandular and respiratory problems reflective of a generalized stress reaction." Workers in particularly noisy environments become increasingly argumentative on the job and at home, show more signs of fatigue, and have more neurotic complaints. Sharp sounds (like sonic booms) cause stress in unborn babies in the womb, city noise levels are constantly rising to create more confusion and stress and deafness and when noise pollution reaches 165 decibels it can kill small animals and terrorize people. We need, as the Bible says, to study to be QUIET.

CARMINATIVES: are herbals having a pungent, warming effect on the stomach, expelling wind and gas, relieving colic and flatulence. These make very fine stomach teas and include such herbs as Allspice, Anise, Caraway, Cardamon, Catnip, Cinnamon bark, Coriander, Cumin seed, Ginger root, Lovage, Mace, Mustard seed, Peppermint leaves, etc. Ginger tea is an old favorite stomach warmer, made from a tablespoonful of the bruised root with a pint of boiling water poured on it and left to stand covered for an hour. Then a tablespoonful or two of the tea is taken at a time. Cayenne Pepper is another carminative.

CATHARTICS: herbal purges and laxatives, include such herbs as Aloes, Agar-agar, Barberry, Blue Flag, Buckthorn bark, Cascara bark, Cassia Fistula, Castor oil, Karaya gum, Manna, Psyllium seed, Rhubarb root, Senna, Tamarind pulp, Coriander seed, and Fennel seed. Care should be exercised in not overdoing it with harsh purges. Once the system is cleaned out, regular eating of fresh fruits and leafy green vegetables will produce a natural, relaxing roughage diet. Helpful also is to take a small glass of warm lemon juice on arising each morning. Any health food store can recommend mild cathartic herb teas. Stay away from harsh, chemical laxatives made of synthetics. Normal, natural elimination prevents many disease complications.

CHOLAGOGUES: are herbals that increase the flow of bile, stimulating the cleansing of the liver and gall bladder. Included here are Wahoo, Fern brake, May apple, Black root, Butternut bark, Oil nut, Water-ash, Culver's root, etc. A German herbal compound called Chola-gutt contains Calamus, Cardui Mariae, Aloes, Chelidonium majus, Lavadula spica, and Peppermint —and I have found this very helpful. But if you suspect a liver or gall condition, consult your doctor or naturopathic practitioner. It is my own personal opinion that many a gall bladder operation could have been avoided with a preventive diet and herbal therapy before it reached the point where the knife was necessary. In the tropics, numerous amebic parasites tend to migrate into the gall and liver ducts and specialists in tropical parasitology should be consulted first to determine whether or not you may have picked up some ameba. Gallstones have reportedly been successfully treated by three different botanicals: either eating raw Blackberries, or homeopathic Belladonna in potency of 200, or use of "Oil of Haarlem" (Dutch Drops). A good preventive is the eating of Leeks. Stone in the bladder has been long treated by Burnet saxifrage and Bladderwrack stewed together in two pints of water for twenty minutes, strained and drunk by the small juice-glassful every three hours, soon dissolving the stones and passing them. Stone in the kidney has been treated by boiling an ounce of Parsley in a pint of water (for an hour) then straining and drinking a small glassful every three hours.

COUNTER-IRRITANTS: herbals causing irritation or mild pain on the body's surface in order to relieve a deeper, more acute pain. Mustard plasters are an example of this type action. VESICANTS or botanicals producing blisters are somewhat of a similar class. The theory is that the minor surface pain ties up the sensory nerves so that the deeper pain cannot get through — this actually works but it remains a question of the complete mechanism involved. Any discussion of counter-irritants is incomplete without reference to some curious, ancient Chinese methods of treatment which are being increasingly accepted nowadays as having many therapeutic merits. One is acupuncture — the practise of inserting small silver needles at various nerve junctures on the surface of the body. The ancient Chinese believed that every organ had channels or "nerve endings" reaching out to specific areas of the skin and that when these were stimulated, an improvement in the organ itself would follow. In 1893 the British neurologist Sir Henry Head discovered that patients suffering from gall bladder or kidney ailments did not necessarily have pains in the afflicted organs but that their pains were referred to certain clearly definable areas of the skin. These zones, even when treated with a simple massage or diathermy (heat treatment) produced a surprisingly beneficial effect. Nowadays they speak of "therapeutic anesthesia", meaning the injection of a local anesthetic in such zones so as to block nerves, causing relief in somatic or visceral pains.

The homeopathic doctor, Dr. Weihe, also discovered 195 skin points having close affinity with the internal organs. The Chinese claim 365 such points. Simple insertion of a needle in the appropriate point is often enough to instantly cause deep internal pain to cease. Why is this? Another Chinese therapy coming into more favor in naturopathic circles today is moxibustion. Pulverized herbs, usually Wormwood, are kneaded into small, cone-shaped lumps, set directly onto the skin zone to be treated, then ignited and left to burn down to the very skin. This cauterization process is also remarkably effective in zone therapy. How exactly it works is a mystery as there is much as yet unknown about the nervous system. Truly we are fearfully and wonderfully made by God! (For more information, consult "CHINESE FOLK MEDICINE", by H. Wallnofer and A. Von Rottauscher, Crown Publishers, Inc., N.Y., 1965, 184 pp.).

The application of external irritants to the skin in order to relieve an internal condition of disease is a practise of great antiquity. Various degrees of irritation may be induced, from the sensation of warmth and reddening of the skin to the stronger blistering action of vesicants and pustulants. Knowledge of the action of counter-irritants is very imperfect. Their most obvious effect, however, is the relief of pain and for this reason they are employed in large numbers of diseases such as gastric disorders, inflammation of the lungs, neuralgia and neuritis. Free organic iodine in solution or in ointment form is a valuable counter-irritant. It is used especially in various forms of arthritis, for the alleviation of acute inflammation, and in glandular enlargement. Its beneficial action has been observed in sciatica and rheumatic diseases. How it works exactly is unknown though no doubt to some extent as a consequence of its being absorbed through the skin. Cinnamon oil is another counter-irritant.

DEMULCENTS: Herbs with a softening effect, sheathing, lubricating internally. They are used to allay irritation of the membranes, coughs and minor throat irritations. They include Agar-agar, Arrow root, Comfrey root, Flaxseed, Gum arabic, Iceland Moss, Irish Moss, Licorice root, Marshmallow root, Okra pods, Oatmeal, Psyllium seed, Sago root, Slippery Elmbark, Tragacanth gum, etc. Herbal teas of these plants can be made from tea bags or mixtures available at your local health food store. It is in place here to discuss especially two of these herbs that have wider therapeutic effects, Licorice and Comfrey. Both have been known since ancient times and tombs of the Egyptian Pharaohs contained large supplies of Licorice, which was not only used as a medicinal herb but to make a sweet, refreshing drink. Licorice is 50 times sweeter than sugar and is one of the few sweets which satisfy thirst instead of arousing it. Licorice is widely used in Europe. the Middle East and China as a blood purifier, demulcent, mild aperient, and expectorant. It is popular in use for sore throats and colds and has been also used as a satisfying substitute for cigarettes by those trying to break the "coffin-nail" habit. Scientific analysis of licorice proved that it contained estrogenic properties and this explains why it has been much used for "female troubles" with success. Who knows what other hormones it might contain? Try chewing it, or drinking licorice water.

Comfrey root has also been used since ancient times specially as a poultice on broken limbs, for ulcers, ugly wounds and burns, tumors and growths. Most of the herbalist writers agree on the wide therapeutic powers of Comfrey. Dr. H. E. Kirschner, in his book "NATURE'S HEALING GRASSES", devotes four chapters to Comfrey. Used internally as a tea made from dried Comfrey roots or leaves, by eating the fresh leaves, or as a fresh juice made from the whole live plant itself, it has been found useful in clearing up long-standing cases of asthma, stomach ulcers, ulcers of the lungs and kidneys, digestive disorders, as a blood purifier in clearing up styes, and a dissolver of phlegm. Because of its effectiveness in promoting healing of broken bones it has been commonly called by the popular name of "Knit-bone". Boneset and Vervain (Verbena) were two other herbal teas used for promoting healing of bone breaks and fractures by the ancients, Externally, used as a poultice, the bruised or macerated leaves of Comfrey have cleared up eczema, skin infections, skin ulcers, rheumatic swellings, skin cancer, breast tumors, second and third degree burns, and promoted rapid healing of fractures and broken bones. Scientific research shows that the Comfrey plant contains two very active healing agents, allantoin and cholin, plus other unknown factors; the allantoin speeds up the formation of new bone cells and skin cells. Since cancer is a disease characterized by the body's cells going haywire and growing abnormally, might it not be found someday that Comfrey's action of promoting normal cell growth could be of great help in fighting cancer? Many claim that Comfrey is helpful in fighting tumors. Most health food stores now stock Comfrey tea, Comfrey dried root poweder or dried leaf powder. The plant is propagated from root cuttings and will grow easily in most gardens.

DEOBSTRUENTS: botanicals that have the effect of clearing obstructions from the natural ducts of the body. This class of herbs includes Common agrimony, Hollyhock, Shepherd's purse, Boneset, and Gravel root. These act upon gall stones and kidney stones. It is appropriate also to mention here that recent medical research has shown a new direction for the clearing of those veins and arteries in the human body that have become clogged with cholesterol like sewer pipes full of grease and sludge. Clogged or blocked blood vessels result in high blood pressure, blood clots, heart breakdowns, etc. When doctors were told that horses with blood clots were successfully treated with a diet of Garlic and Onions, they investigated the effects on patients with blood clots, having them eat quantities of pure fat accompanied by onions (fried, boiled or raw). In every case the anti-clotting factors in the blood rose as the Onions seemed to cancel out or dissolve the fats. Research is now going on to see what factors in the Onion and Garlic accomplish this. It has long been known that Garlic lowers high blood pressure. Presumably something in its volatile oil helps to clean out fatty wastes, dilate the blood vessels, etc.

Those of us who live in the tropics and must be on guard against the contamination of drinking water by such parasites as amebas, have been glad to discover a sensible and inexpensive system of automatically injecting organic iodine into the water supply in minute quantities. The iodine does not injure the body at all but kills every known type of virus and ameba. Furthermore, iodine medication has a definite deobstruent action on the body, driving out impurities from the blood and tissues. Internal iodine medication has a salutary effect on thyroid diseases such as goiter, amebic dysentery, and even on such respiratory diseases as asthma, bronchitis, flu, catarrh and the common cold. High doses of iodine administered externally have a disinfectant, alterative, and counter-irritant value, as mentioned previously. Internal, deobstruent action is also seen with iodine affecting arteriosclerosis and diseases of circulation. An ancient deobstruent that has been recently revived as a health food is common sea-weed or Kelp. Old time herbalists used it in treatment of obesity and goiter as well as for many other ailments. Each year thousands of tons of Kelp are now being harvested in the U.S. and turned into food supplements, medicines, health foods and cattle feeds. Kelp is especially rich in organic iodine plus many other vital trace minerals.

Iodine is necessary for the thyroid gland's proper performance of its work. All the blood in the body passes through the thyroid gland every 17 minutes and its concentration of iodine kills germs. But the thyroid gland's iodine content is dependent on the iodine available in the food and water intake of a person. Iodine acts as an inner germ killer, reliever of nervous tension (a malfunctioning thyroid causes hyperactive nervousness), and assists clear thinking. A good supplement to your diet is to drink daily a glass of water containing one drop of Lugol's solution of Iodine (available at your drugstore), one ounce of apple cider vinegar, and two teaspoonfuls of honey. Honey has many wonderful medicinal qualities and both it and the apple cider vinegar are beneficial in correcting constipation and aiding arthritis conditions. Drink 20 minutes before a meal.

DIAPHORETICS: are those herbal substances having the effect of producing mild perspiration; SUDORIFICS are in the same category but stimulate abundant perspiration. When it is understood that the body needs to pass off its wastes not only through excretion and urine but also through sweat, it will be readily understood how important these medicines are. In the Bible it is recorded that God commanded Adam: "In the sweat of thy face shalt thou eat bread" (Genesis 3:19) and woe unto the man who does not labor enough to pass wastes off from his body by sweat. Experiments have shown that people whose sweat glands have been blocked, by painting the skin over the whole surface of the body with some impermeable substance, will soon sicken and die because of the accumulation of toxic wastes. Any approach to systemic healing (treating the whole system of the sick person rather than merely an isolated symptom or two), should include steam bath therapy to begin a thorough "house cleaning". Producing copious sweating from the use of internal medication is possible too and the following are generally herbs used for this: Elder flowers, Goose grass, Burdock root, Peppermint leaves, Sage leaves, Yarrow, Tansy, Anise, Blessed Thistle, Horsemint, Canada snake root, German Chamomile, Pleurisy root, Hoarhound, etc. Sudorifics (stronger than Diaphoretics): Ague Weed herb, Ginger root,

Hyssop herb, Pennyroyal, Serpentaria root, Crawley root, Boneset, Blue Cohosh, and Mayweed. These are generally taken as a hot tea before retiring. (Incidentally for bedwetting children, try a spoonful of honey on retiring — it acts as a moisture retentive as well as a calmative).

DIURETICS: are herbs that increase the secretion and flow of urine. Never forget that water taken internally flushes the system and aids the elimination of wastes; taken externally it is both healing and soothing. For thousands of years mankind has been repairing to health spas to drink and bathe in waters with high mineral content. The chief curative mineral in most famous spas is magnesium sulphate (Epsom salts) and one can have a good mineral bath at home by adding a good double handful of Epsom salts to the ordinary hot water bath. The action of the salts is to draw out the acids and if one continually keeps rubbing the body and limbs while in the bath, better action is produced. One need only remain in the water for four or five minutes; use no soap during the mineral bath. Rheumatic sufferers and those with arthritis, lumbago, etc., should take an Epsom salt bath twice weekly. Concerning the diuretic herbs, they include: Bearberry or Uva Ursi leaves, Bilberry leaves, Broom tops, Burdock seeds, Couch grass, Cubeb berries, Juniper berries, Copaiba Balsam, Gravel plant, Princess Pine leaves, Parsley root, Watermelon seed, Elecampane root, Corn silk, Dog grass root, and many others. Especially the Bearberry leaves are a good diuretic and like the others may be made up into a hot tea. Caution should be observed to use diuretics sparingly so as not to exhaust the kidneys by abuse. But many urinary and kidney disturbances respond to treatment with diuretic teas.

Dropsy, or the accumulation of excess fluids in the tissues, is treated with such herbals as Broom tea with the occasional addition of Queen of the Meadow, Dandelion root, American Mandrake, Greater Celandine, Horehound, etc., stewed together in three quarts of water for twenty minutes, strained when cool and then drunk in the quantity of about 4 ounces three times daily. For external treatment, a lump of camphor is dissolved into an 8 ounce bottle full of methylated spirits (wintergreen) and rubbed on the spot night and morning. Gout is another tricky disease accompanied by a high uric acid level in the body. Foods like sweetbreads, kidney, liver, sardines, anchovies and gravy extracts must be avoided. Herbs increasing the urinary output of uric acid are most helpful. Homeopathically, gout is often treated with Nux vomica 6, or Urtica urens, or Pulsatilla alternated with Acon. Parsley tea or fresh-pressed Parsley juice is a good diuretic. Also cucumber juice added to carrot and beet juice is beneficial in rheumatic ailments resulting from the excessive uric acid in the system — good for flushing out the gall bladder, liver, kidneys and prostrate glands. One or two pints of this combation of juices should be taken daily, while also cutting down on flour, sugar, and meat in the diet.

Once again we find our old friend Garlic is an effective agent here as a diuretic, as well as having a strengthening and slightly laxative effect. Numerous seeds have diuretic properties and there has been a renewed interest in the nutritional and medicinal benefits of eating seeds. Anise seed is widely valued as a diuretic, Caraway seed for an upset stomach and gas, Celery seed for rheumatism, Burdock seed tea as a blood purifier and cleanser to eliminate styes and boils, Sunflower seeds and Soybean seeds are richest in vitamin B factors, Carrot seed extract is used to stimulate animal fertility, Pumpkin seeds are widely used to kill worms and benefit prostrate gland disorders (besides being diuretic they seem to rejuvenate the prostrate gland), Sesame seeds and Safflower seeds seem to be valuable aids in preventing cholesterol from collecting in the blood. Recently there has been also a great interest in juices pressed and drunk fresh from sprouted seeds. Experiments have shown the sprouting wheat seeds, corn seeds and rice and bean seeds are tremendously richer in concentrated vitamins and anti-biotics than the mature plant or the mere seed itself. It seems that during germination more vitamins are produced and the fresh pressed juice of the sprouts is powerful. For thousands of years the Chinese have recognized and used the tremendous values of bean sprouts and bamboo shoots and other early plant stages. Many nowadays are drinking wheat grass juice and finding it very beneficial. Try eating some of these above-mentioned seeds which have such a salutary effect on urino-genitary disorders. Most any large grocery store stocks most of these seeds in the spice section. Try juicing and eating fresh seed sprouts. You can sprout your own in trays set in the windows of your own home. Metal pans are recommended to be used (but not aluminum or plastic) and seeds that are not treated with insecticides should be used, naturally. Mulch under the roots back into the soil after you have "harvested" the young shoots (when several inches high) for eating or juicing.

EMETICS: are herbs that cause vomiting. There are many of these type herbs that are used in weaker solutions for other, more beneficial purposes but in large doses or strong concenations have a violent vomitory effect. One might wonder what possible good purpose that vomiting could serve but a moment's thought will remind us that accidental poisoning can be sometimes neutralized by provoking vomiting to rid the stomach of the poison. The herb Ipecac is used as an emergency specific to cause vomiting in cases of poisoning (however, if strychnine or corrosives such as lye, strong acids, petroleum distillates such as kerosene, gasoline, coal oil, fuel oil, paint thinner or cleaning fluid have been ingested, Ipecac is not used because vomiting would just spread the poisons through the lungs, etc. In such cases, something like Unidote — Universal Antidote containing activated charcoal, magnesium oxide and tannic acid — is used as it absorb or neutralizes the poisons. Immediate first aid with herbals is appropriate as discussed but remember that the doctor should be notified at once in all cases of poisoning and the patient rushed to the hospital where stomach pumps and other helps are available.

Other common emetics are Dogbane, Swamp milkweed, Blessed thistle, Scotch broom, Wild Yam or Colic root, Boneset, Ilex Cassina, Blue Flag, Vervain, Lobelia, etc. Taking these emetics can be dangerous and should be undertaken only under direction of a physician or naturopathic practitioner. The gluttonous ancient Romans used emetics for a very frivolous purpose — it was customary in wealthy homes to have a room beside the dining room, called the vomitorium, and after grossly indulging in food and drink, they staggered out to the vomitorium and with emetics spewed forth the contents of their stomachs so that they could glut themselves again! Other ancient peoples sometimes practised vomiting with emetics in order to purify the stomach and system.

EMOLLIENTS: herbs having a softening effect, causing warmth, moisture; lotions or ointments for the skin. These include agents generally of an oily or mucilaginous nature, used externally, such as Comfrey root (already discussed under Demulcents), Flaxseed meal (—incidentally, an old remedy for something irritating the eye-ball is to place a small flax seed under the eye-lid and it swells up into a mucilaginous mass attracting the irritant to itself and can then be easily removed), Marshmallow leaves or root, oatmeal, Quince seed, Slippery Elm bark, etc. Nivea skin cream is a German product including many old herbal ingredients and can be purchased in your local drug-store. A simple lotion for chapped skin can be made of four parts of olive oil to one part of white wax. For fresh burns and scalds the Scotch use Carron Oil— one part limewater to two parts Flaxseed or Cottonseed oil. Modern medical science is here again returning to an age-old remedy as the latest opinion is that merely simple, cold water is the best first aid treatment for burns! (Over wide areas, cloths soaked in cold water should be applied until the patient arrives at the hospital — this will retard loss of vital fluids and cool and soothe the hurt). You can concoct your own favorite ointments simply at home by taking a base of some petroleum jelly like Vaseline and melting it down to mix with herbal oils. Cocoa butter, easily purchased in your local drug store, is one of the best soothing oitments for chapped skin, sunburns, abrasions, dry skin, etc. In olden times, honey and almond was a favorite mix for hand lotions. (Other interesting creams and lotions are discussed in Gayelord Hauser's "TREASURY OF SECRETS", Fawcett Publications, Inc., 1966, 576 pp. and in "NATURAL BEAUTY SECRETS", by Deborah Rutledge, Avon Books, 1967, 166 pp.). A refreshing emollient bath can be made at home by combining one cup of olive oil with 1 tablespoon of any liquid detergent shampoo and one teaspoon of oil of Rose Geranium (available at your drug store). Shake vigorously each time before using and put two tablespoons of the mixture into your tub full of warm water. Witch Hazel is also soothing for sun burn. Scented olive oil was much used in Roman baths. Using olive oil was the main media for transferring scents from herbs, flowers and spices in ancient times.

EXPECTORANTS: these are herbs that stimulate the secretion of saliva, spitting, and the expulsion of phlegm. They are often combined with demulcents to make cough medicines. Incidentally, a wonderful cough syrup is Syrupus Pini Albae Compositus (Compound White Pine Cough Syrup). It contains not only White pine bark but also Wild cherry bark, Spikenard, Poplar buds, Bloodroot, Sassafrass, and Amaranth. Common expectorants are: Balsam of Tolu, Benzoin, Coltsfoot, Hoarhound, Elecampane, Blood root, Ipecac (see caution under Emetics), Licorice root, Wild Ginger, Wild Cherry bark, Comfrey, Pleurisy root, Yerba Santa, etc.

FEBRIFUGES: see ANTIPYRETICS, treating fevers.

FUNGICIDALS: herbs tending to kill fungicidal infections. The root of the Pokewood (Phytolacca) applied externally is an old ringworm remedy. The common Burdock (Arctium) is an old- fashioned remedy for psoriasis. Witch hazel is still a popular remedy for itching skin, mild sun burn, and poison ivy rash (when mixed with equal parts of baking soda to make a paste). Stubborn cases of eczema have been cured by taking homeopathic pills containing Sulphur, Apis and Rhus Tox, all in potencies of 200. Eczema is a symptom of impurities in the blood and so has to be got at from within. A powerful antidote for many kinds of fungus and also for alleviating cases of ivy poisoning is Jewelweed or Touch-me-not. A quantity boiled down until the juice is concentrated is very effective for washing off the areas afflicted with ivy poison (it is also useful to wash with after having been exposed to poison ivy or even before any rash has appeared, as a preventive). A salve prepared from Jewelweed plants boiled with lard is reputed to help cure piles; the raw juice will remove warts and corns and cure ringworm, according to Potter's "CYCLO PEDIA OF BOTANICAL DRUGS AND PREPARATIONS." Athlete's foot is also killed by it.

Since the disasters that have followed upon indiscriminate use of hard pesticides like D.D.T. which persist in the ground and environment and kill and damage long after they have been applied, more emphasis is being put now on finding and using organic fungicides and insecticides. If you do not wish to expose your family to chemical poisoning and yet wish to kill the insects look around for a NON-TOXIC TO HUMANS OR PETS label on an insecticide and note that it is probably compounded from the Pyrethrum plant (deadly to all insects but harmless to warm-blooded creatures). Nature is an incomparable store-house of God-given remedies! Oil of Citronella rubbed on exposed areas of the skin will repel insects. Oil of lavender sprayed lightly throughout a bookcase will save leather bindings from mold, according to an old recipe. Garlic oil kills mosquito larvae.

The U.S. government is so concerned (finally!) about the persistence of hard pesticides (D.D.T., aldrin, dieldrin, endrin, heptachlor, benzene hexachloride, lindane and arsenic, lead or mercury compounds) that they are taking steps to phase out their use. However, so much has already polluted the soil, gone into the streams and down into the ocean, that it is estimated that every man, woman and child in the U.S. is carrying a minute quantity of D.D.T. in their bodies, wild-life are dying from it, fish are dying, and D.D.T. is even found in the tissues of living creatures in Antarctica — none of it was ever sprayed there but it has leached out and spread down there through the oceans. A shocking fact is that mentioned by the January 26, 1970 NEWSWEEK magazine: "American women carry in their breasts milk that has anywhere from three to ten times more of the pesticide D.D.T. than the Federal government allows in dairy milk meant for human consumption." Each year 200 million tons of smoke and fumes, including millions of tons of poisonous exhaust, metal particles, noxious oils and chemicals, is belched out into the American skies and falls down like a rain of death on the land. Air pollution is killing pine trees as far as 60 miles away from Los Angeles! Most metropolitan areas average 15,000 particles of air pollution per cubic centimeter of air now and it is increasing at the rate of 1,500 per year; the pollution level will be deadly for humans at 35,000 particles and it is expected this will be reached in the early 1980's! Proposals are being studied to cover the cities with domes or instruct the populace in wearing gas masks in the forseeable future. Noxious industrial and automobile exhaust fumes are causing a tremendous upswing in asthma, bronchitis, lung cancer and emphysema. A man need not even smoke cigarettes to get lung cancer now — he just needs to live in a heavily polluted area and breathe in the poisons. Air pollution, soil pollution, water pollution — man in his folly is poisoning his environment with his modern, get-rich-quick inventions. Man cannot poison nature without in the long run poisoning himself. Yet they continue to use enormous quantities of pesticides and herbicides in order to "more efficiently" produce the food crops we are eating! The cattle we use for meat are fed on powerful synthetic drugs and hormones — with the caution that they are not to be used for food until 30 days have elapsed after their last "treatment", but who can be sure these "cautions" are observed? The processed foods we are offered in the super-markets invariably have been treated with food additives and preservatives containing powerful chemicals and when one type, the cyclamates, was recently declared cancer-causing by the U.S. government and announcement made that all foods containing this additive must be off the market by February, 1970, commercial interests raised such a howl that the government back-pedalled and gave more time to sell them off to the innocent consumers! The Surgeon General's office has warned that cigarettes can cause cancer but the efforts to discourage their sales are very feeble and ineffective because it is a market earning billions of dollars! The profit in poisons is tremendous AND SO IS THE RISING DEATH RATE FROM THEM! Man's indiscriminate use of powerful chemical fertilizers, pesticides and herbicides to produce his crops has caused more than one person to think it might be better to desist from such types of crop production and eat the safer weeds (HERBS) which he is trying to kill off with his herbicides! Until recently, the sea itself was looked upon as a great potential source of natural food but recent news releases say that the Kelp beds are dying off the coasts of "civilized countries" and the sea itself becoming polluted with oil, scum, garbage, poisons, etc. When will man learn?

LAXATIVES: herbs which stimulate mild evacuation of the intestines and bowels; see the section on APERIENTS for milder laxatives and the section on CATHARTICS for stronger laxatives. These include Cascara bark, Golden Seal, Senna pods, Gentian, Yellow Root, Butternut bark, Turtlebloom, Licorice root, Dandelion root, and Peach Tree leaves. A tea can be made from any of these with a teaspoonful to a cup of boiling water. Allow to cool and drink a small dose once a day. When normal evacuations are regained, discontinue using a laxative. If stronger doses are taken hot, and more frequently, naturally results will be more violent.

NERVINES: herbals which tend to strengthen the nerves, relax tension temporarily and relieve nervous strain and fatigue. They include Asafetida gum, Betony herb, Catnip herb, Chamomile flowers, Hops flowers, Lettuce leaves and juice, Nerve root, Passion flower, Scullcap herb, Skunk cabbage root, Valerian root, Yarrow herb, Mistletoe, Lady Slipper. Compound your own tea out of a few ounces of several of these or secure a ready-mixed compound nervine tea from your health food store. As Christianity declines in our modern world, nervous tension increases. A Christian approach to a real mental problem will do far more than months and years of psycho-analysis in most cases. Nerves, like any other part of the body, become irritable and overwrought if one is living at a tense, fearful, unnatural pace. Why worry when you can pray?

NARCOTICS: are powerful, dangerous herbal or chemical drugs bringing illusory feeling of well-being by depressing cretain nerve centers. Marijuana, opium and its derivatives (morphine and heroine), coca and cocaine, alcohol, peyotl (mescaline), kava, betel, to say nothing of LSD and all the other synthetics — these generally all contain powerful alkaloids which intoxicate the nervous system and tend to become habit-forming and finally addictive. One pays a terribly high price for experimenting with such things and becoming a slave of them. Yearly hundreds and thousands of people become living robots through drug slavery. The wisdom of herbalism and homeopathy is in its limitation of dosages of even the beneficial herbs. Even something beneficial can become a poison in overdoses. Anyone making his own herbal tea from plants that he has collected himself had better know his stuff as some herbs are so potent they will kill. An Idaho sheepherder was found dead surrounded by his dead flock. The sheep had been eating a harmless looking little white flower called the "Death Camas". The shepherd had eaten meat from one of the sheep and had been poisoned himself.

Other poisonous plants, unless properly diluted, are the Lily-of-the-Valley root (a medicinal heart stimulant), Jimsonweed or Thorn apple (containing an anodyne), and Henbane (a sedative). The philosopher Socrates was executed by an annoyed government through being sentenced to drink Hemlock (no relation to the evergreen tree by that name but a poisonous biennial herb whose leaves look like Parsley). Some plants are relatively harmless to animals but deadly to man — like the White Flowering Snakeroot which can be eaten by cattle without harm but then renders their milk fatally poisonous to man (the mother of Abraham Lincoln died of milk poisoning in 1818 when Abe was 9 years old). Avoid all narcotics like the plague; eat no herbs or plants that you are not sure are harmless. Yearly billions of dollars and thousands of lives are wasted in the tragedy of narcotics addiction. Without mentioning the tragedy of alcoholism, even tobacco, coffee, chocolate and ordinary commercial tea contain habit-forming stimulants which harm millions of people by making them dependent. The Bible warns against becoming the slave of anything.

The February 2, 1970 TIME magazine, in a feature article on pollution of the environment, points out that just as people get hooked on drugs, so the soil seems to become addicted to chemical additives and loses its ability to fix its own nitrogen and as a result more and more fertilizer has to be used until it has now reached the stage where nitrates are turning up in the water supply, endangering human health. But to wean farmers away from pesticides and chemical fertilizers would cause at least a temporary decline in farm productivity and a hike in food prices; ecologists are recommending return to organic fertilizers, crop rotation, and control of insect pests by fighting them with their insect enemies. The use of DDT has killed off the birds that eat up the insects and also produced DDT-resistant insects! Man has poisoned his environment AND HIMSELF; like a species of filth-eating vulture, he has befouled his own nest. Along with air pollution, soil pollution, and water pollution, man has fallen victim to spreading plagues of degenerative diseases like cancer, heart-trouble and insanity — a poisoned heritage of chemical pesticides, herbicides, food additives, fertilizers and automobile and industrial wastes and gases. And how does man try to conquer these chemical-induced or aggravated diseases? Of course, he turns to powerful, synthetic chemical drugs with unpredictable side effects! It will be a great awakening medically when the many people who are concerned about using organic fertilizer for their crops wake up to using organic medicines for their own bodies instead of the synthetic drugs.

PECTORAL: herbals useful in diseases of the lung or chest. The reader may wish to refer also to the section on Expectorants, as they are often used in combination with Pectorals to loosen phlegm, dry up catarrh, and fight coughs. Hoarhound is widely used in cough drops, as are also Wild Cherry bark, Menthol (mint extracts), etc. Wild Ginger-root, Spikenard, Poplar buds, Blood root, Sassafrass root bark, Amaranth, and others are used as Pectorals. Our old friends Garlic, Onion and Ginseng are often found as ingredients in home remedies for asthma, bronchitis, coughs, colds and hoarseness. Some herbals recommend Syrup of Garlic, made by pouring a quart of boiling water on a pound of fresh Garlic cut into slices, allowing it to stand thus for twelve hours in a closed vessel then open and add honey to make it the consistency of syrup; a little Caraway and Sweet Fennel seed bruised and boiled for a short time in vinegar and then added to the Syrup of Garlic will cover its pungent smell. Another interesting item tying Garlic, Onion and Ginseng root together is the discovery by a Russian electrobiologist, Professor Gurwith, that a peculiar type of ultra-violet radiation called mitogenetic radiation was found to be emitted by all three. These radiations had the property of stimulating cell growth and activity in Onions, Garlic and Ginseng. It is supposed that these radiations might have a rejuvenating effect on body cells in general but especially on the sexual and other endocrine glands. Numerous hormones have been found active in these powerful herbs as well. Many mysteries remain unexplained in the complex make-up of even such simple herbs and vegetables. If the volatile oils of these herbs contain the active substances, as is quite likely, then treatment of respiratory ailments by inhalation would be a powerfully effective therapy. (See the section on Aromatics). We know that Onions and Garlic, and possibly also Ginseng, were used in Bible times for medicinal purposes. In Ezekiel 27:17 we read that "they traded in thy market wheat of Minnith, and Pannag (Ginseng?), and honey, and oil and balm."

POULTICES: are a soft mass of crushed plant matter applied to the surface of the body. The Bible mentions one such poultice specifically: "And Isaiah said, Take a lump (poultice) of figs. And they took and laid it on the boil, and (king Hezekiah) recovered." (II. Kings 20:7). We have already referred to the Old Testament king Solomon, of whom it was said he was the author of 39 books in his lifetime, one of them a book on the medicinal qualities of plants and trees. Unfortunately, this book has been lost although what may be a reference to it is found in I. Kings 4:33 — "And he (Solomon) spake of trees, from the cedar tree that is in Lebanon even unto the hyssop that springeth up out of the wall..." How wonderful it would be if we could read Solomon's own herbal book! Nonetheless, God's book of Nature still stands, open for all who desire to study and discover what is there. Poultices have been used from time immemorial for healing. We have previously referred to two of the most powerful kinds of herbal poultices: Comfrey and Garlic.

As the Comfrey leaves contain little juice but rather a thick, mucilaginous substance, the leaves are usually macerated or bruised until gooey, then spread on a cloth and tied over the infected area. As the roots of Comfrey also contain allantoin, the principal therapeutic property, they may be crushed in the poultice too. Comfrey poultices have been used on ulcers, wounds, infections, over broken limbs, bad burns, skin cancers, etc. Dried Comfrey powder can be used for poultices if the fresh leaves are not available. Garlic poultices can be made by removing the outer shells from the small cloves of Garlic, chopping them finely, and making enough ready to be ¼ inch deep and cover the soles of each foot; first grease the soles with vaseline then tie on the poultice with thin linen. Cover the feet and poultice with an old sock at night so it will not fall off. This is a remedy reputed very good for whooping cough in children. Garlic poultices are also used on the chest for bad colds and pneumonia, on ulcers and wounds, and on rheumatic inflammations. For treating warts, try a poultice of juice from the May apple root or also lemon rinds soaked for 24 hours in vinegar and applied with the white inner rind of the lemon to the wart for three hours, then re-applied freshly every three hours. The Violet plant was used as far back as 500 B.C. in poultice form as a reputed cure for surface cancers. It is used in England and some parts of the U.S. for the same purpose even today.

Other useful poultices include the Bran poultice (a flannel or linen bag is filled loosely with Bran, placed in a bowl and boiling water poured over it — after soaking well, it is then removed, wrung out in a towel to remove excess water, and then it is applied as hot as can be stood on the painful place (such as in neuritis, neuralgia, synovitis, sciatica, spinal pains, abdominal upset, etc.). The poultice is covered with dry material and allowed to stay on until cold. Another is the herb poultice — fill a linen bag with Chamomile or Hops or equal parts of both and proceed as in the Bran poultice. Then there is the Linseed poultice — moisten a small quantity of Linseed with boiling water in a basin, stir thoroughly, spread to a thickness of about ½ inch on linen and apply as hot as possible; this is reportedly good for bronchitis, coughs, asthma and pneumonia. For respiratory troubles, the poultice should cover the whole chest and remain on for two hours. Slippery Elm poultice is made by mixing powdered Slippery Elm with Oatmeal or Barley Flour, mixed with hot water and spread over linen to be applied hot; the Potato poultice is made from scraped, raw Potatoes applied on linen and used cold on septic wounds. All of the above hot poultices should be followed by washing the skin down after the poultice is removed with a mix of ½ vinegar and ½ water to prevent skin discoloration. Some use hot salt (heated on a tray and placed in a bag) for toothache, neuralgia and neuritis. Clove oil temporarily lessens toothache (until you can see your dentist). In a severe toothache, clean out the cavity then insert a plug of cotton saturated with Oil of Capsicum and it will in most cases cure the toothache by its stimulating and antiseptic qualities. The effect is reputed to last for months. However, common sense will tell you that toothaches come from decay and fermentation working in cavities and the best solution in the long run is to have the dentist clean out and fill the cavities.

PURGATIVES: herbs that promote abundant and frequent evacuations of the bowels. These have a stronger action than ordinary cathartics and the mild aperients and should be used sparingly and seldom. Constantly taking purgatives cannot cure; in time they so weaken the bowels that a natural movement is impossible. An occasional enema is better than taking purgatives. They include Buckthorn bark, Black root, Butternut bark, Mayapple root, Boneset herb, Senna leaves. The ancients used to use purgatives sparingly and in cases of extreme blockage; the American Indians used purgatives in the spring of the year as a kind of spring house-cleaning. Autopsies performed on many cadavers have proved over and over again that the modern city dweller often dies with his intestines full of dried, hardened fecal matter that may have been the cause of auto-intoxication and the stimulus for many fatal diseases. Chronic constipation has been cured by diet alone. A glass of warm water with Lemon juice before breakfast, prunes soaked in warm water, "All-bran" or other roughage cereals, taking a short, sharp walk before breakfast, abdominal massage, these all stimulate normal bowel movements. Sufferers should remember that the natural position for evacuation is a squat rather than the seated position; the native squat squeezes the abdomen and distends the back passage. Native peoples rarely suffer from constipation until they become "civilized" and adopt poor foods and chair-toilets.

REFRIGERANTS: herbs with a cooling effect, lowering body heat. They include the following, from which delicious teas and refreshing cool drinks may be made for hot weather: Boneset herb, Goose grass, Peruvian bark, Gravel plant, Borage herb, Licorice root, Melissa herb, Pimpernel herb, Raspberry fruit, Tamarind pulp, Yerba Santa leaves, Balm. Refreshing drinks made from these herbs are much superior to carbonated soft drinks loaded with gas, artificial flavorings and colorings, harmful sugar substitutes, etc.

RUBEFACIENTS: herbs that have the effect of reddening the surface of the skin or lining of a hollow organ by attracting blood to that area. These are very similar in action to Counter-irritants, only much milder. They include Water plantain, Garlic, Wintergreen, Pennyroyal, Prickly pear, Rue, Hemlock spruce, Slippery Elm, and Mullein. This latter is sometimes called "Quaker rouge" for a quaint reason; Quaker girls (like most Plain People) had been taught not to use cosmetics nor to paint their faces yet they early learned that by rubbing a Mullein leaf on their cheeks, extra blood would flow to that area and give the cheeks a rosy glow! Rubefacients are all herbs that will induce such skin surface reddening. It is not advisable to rub Prickly pear on your cheeks as you will produce more than a glow! In weaker dilutions, many rubefacients are just astringent in action. An old recipe for banishing warts says to try rubbing the wart about 20 times daily with Castor oil. Papaya juice rubbed on warts is also reputed to remove them. One of the best liniments for rheumatism or bruises and aches is reportedly made by boiling gently for ten minutes one tablespoonful of Cayenne Pepper in one pint of cider vinegar, then bottling hot, unstrained.

SEDATIVES: have the effect of depressing, calming, tranquilizing the vital powers. These herbals exert a soothing and quieting influence but do not have narcotic effects (see the comments on Calmatives and Narcotics). Peach Tree leaves, Wild Cherry bark, Goose grass, Catnip leaves, Hop flowers, Wild Bull Nettle, Black Cohosh root, Black Haw bark, Chamomile flowers, Motherwort herb, Cramp bark, Squaw weed, and Yarrow herb, are all sedative in action. The same cautions made concerning Calmatives apply equally here.

SOPORIFICS: are herbals producing and conducive to better, deeper sleep. They include Cowslip, Hops (stuffed inside the pillow they induce relaxed sleep), Ladies' Slipper, Lime Flowers (used in bed-time baths to overcome insomnia), Scullcap, Valerian, and Lettuce. A surprisingly simple and efective soporific for those who sleep badly from overstrain is the eating of fresh Lettuce leaves to induce a deeper, more relaxed normal sleep. For ages Orientals have applied Nutmeg oil to their temples as an aid to induce sleep. Warm Elder Berry juice, drunk when retiring, promotes deep natural sleep. Honey taken before retiring is a soporific. Bees are real herbalists, collecting from millions of flowers to make one pound of honey!

STIMULATIVES: herbs exciting the vital powers and nerves. The action of stimulatives tends to be immediate, powerful, but transitory

Common herbal stimulants include Anise, Balm, Cinnamon, Clove, Dill Seed, Cayenne Pepper (one of the best), Elecampane, Ginger, Golden Rod, Horseradish, Hyssop, Savory, Spearmint, Lavender, Marjoram, Nutmeg, Peppermint, etc. They are usually drunk in the form of teas brewed from the fresh or dried herbs or inhaled as vapors from the volatile oils. When depressed or exhausted from a hard day's work the best refreshment is normal sleep; many exhaust their nervous system by trying to repair overwork and tension with stimulants instead of rest. Coffee and commercial tea contain, respectively, powerful stimulative elements known as caffeine and theine (and tannin) and are better left for use as an occasional medicine rather than a daily habit which may burden the nerves. A cold morning shower is an excellent means of stimulating the whole nervous system. The ancients used hot baths followed by cold as stimulants. A hot shower followed by a brief cold shower and a vigorous friction rub-down with a volatile oil like Eucalyptus is very stimulating. If you live in a cold climate, try a Finnish bath (steam bath followed by friction of herbs or pine needles or birch branches against the skin and then a roll in the snow — this is guaranteed to bring a glow to the body!). It should be mentioned here that one of the greatest pieces of misinformation about smoking is that it is supposed to be a stimulant — actually it is a depressant. Tobacco and its smoke contains over 28 poisons and must be classed as a dangerous narcotic; it has been asserted on good evidence that cigarette smoking kills up to 300,000 people a year, yet it remains a multi-billion dollar annual business.

STOMACHICS: tonics stimulating and strengthening the stomach and appetite. See the section on Bitter Tonics. Comfrey tea is a good stomachic, as are also Baya Maté, Golden Seal, Gentian, Wild Ginger, Wild Strawberry, Blackberry root, Uva Ursi leaves, and Pleurisy root. In our affluent society, loss of appetite is seldom met with in comparison with glutted appetites, surfeiting and feasting, and obesity. Many are under the delusion that obesity (overweight) is a sign of health when in reality it is usually always simply a sickness. The accumulation of fat and grease in the body is the source of many illnesses. Curative plants which will help cut down and correct that obese person's appetite are the following — a good recipe calls for equal parts of all the following combined in one teaspoonful per cup, three cups to be drunk daily: Agar-agar, Dandelion leaves and roots, Broom, Buckthorn bark and berries, Chicory, Buckbean (Marsh Trefoil). Some plants that are an aid to fat reduction will also ennable the very thin to put on weight, such as Kelp; because it is rich in iodine and helps normalize the action of the thyroid gland, Kelp can often reduce obesity due to glandular imbalance. If it is inconvenient to obtain the plant in crude form, Homeopathic Fucus (the botanic name for Kelp) in potency of 30, five pills dissolved on the tongue morning and night for three or four weeks may be tried. Naturally one must also cut down intake of starches, fats and sweet drinks. To sweeten bad breath, chew Cardamon seed, Star Anise, Nutmegs, or Cloves after a meal.

STYPTICS: herbals checking or stopping bleeding. They include Puffball, Persimmon, Alum root, Mock pennyroyal, White walnut, Self-heal (Prunella vulgaris), Scarlet sumac, Cup plant and Skunk cabbage. For nose bleeding, a small cotton wad saturated with Witch hazel (or with Calendula lotion) and pushed well up into the nostril will bring quick relief. Homeopathic Phosphorus pilules reputedly swiftly stop bleeding, even after tooth extraction. Homeopathic Crotalus horridus 30 has the same effect. An old remedy often used for internal bleeding is to stew an ounce of Comfrey root in a pint of water for 20 minutes, strain, and give a half cupful about ¼ hour before each meal. Bleeding wounds are treated with homeopathic Calendula lotion, neat, applied to the wound. Naturally, common first aid measures should be taken such as using the pressure points to stop any extensive bleeding, then rush patient to hospital.

SUDORIFICS: are herbs producing abundant perspiration or sweating. They include Horsemint, Mayweed, Blue Cohosh, Boneset, Sage leaves, Wild Ginger, Jamaica Ginger and Crawley root. Steam baths are a good mechanical sudorific especially when accompanied by vapor from aromatic oils of the above plants. The sweat produced by hard work is the most healthful! However, a general house cleaning with a steam bath is salutary from time to time. (See Diaphoretics). Beware of harsh chemical antiperspirants sold to prevent underarm sweating.

THORACIC: herbs used to treat complaints of the lungs and bronchial tubes. See Pectorals.

TRANQUILIZERS: herbs having a calmative effect; see Calmatives.

VERMIFUGES: herbs destroying and expelling worms. See Antihelmintics.

VULNERARIES: herbal washes, sprays, douches (external and internal), etc. The following have been used for many centuries. All-Heal herb, Fleabane, Calendula, Golden Seal, Violet leaves, Plantain leaves, Comfrey, Horse Tail grass, White Oak bark, Slippery Elm, Centauria, Chickweed, etc. See Astringents and Antiseptics. A friend from Oregon, Mr. Frank Kropf, reports that a combination of garlic oil and vinegar is very good for washing out and disinfecting wounds.

Mr. Loren Ross of Santa Ana, Costa Rica, reports that natives tap the sap from the roots of the Guinea Negro Banana tree as a drink in treating patients suffering from hepatitis.

CHAPTER VII:—Live Foods That Are Also Herbal Medicines:

Since first writing this book on the healing powers of God-given herbs, I have made an extensive study of the medicinal qualities found in many common foods. I am taking this opportunity of the need of another printing of this book to include in it virtually an entire, new chapter on this subject of the medicinal qualities inherent in various foods. So important is the subject of proper nutrition, and yet so generally neglected and mis-understood in our times, that I felt strongly there was room for an entire book on this subject alone and accordingly I have written a new book, entitled BIO-NUTRONICS: THE SCIENCE OF LIVE NU-TRITIONAL THERAPY. The book on Bio-Nutronics is a sequel to this book on herbs and yet some of the information is so closely related that it must be included partially in this new chapter. In this brief space it will be impossible to go into great detail so for those who may be vitally interested in the science of therapeutic nutrition, I can only refer you to the more extensive treatment of this subject in my new book on BIO-NUTRONICS.

Biochemically, we are what we eat. Very simply, this means that our physical and mental health is dependent on what kinds of chemicals we put into our bodies. Bio-chemicals or living chemicals from live foods are the best diet to feed and sustain our body chemistry. Live foods heal as well as nourish the body but dead, processed or contaminated foods tend to constipate, hinder and even poison the natural body processes. The father of medicine, Hippocrates, thousands of years ago formulated two fundamental principles of healing: 1. "Your food shall be your medicine, and your medicine shall be your food." 2. "Leave your drugs in the chemist's pot if you can heal the patient with food." Just as herbs are truly foods that act as medicines, so live plant foods are an essential part of the God-given herbs designed by our Creator to heal our ills.

THE BIO-CHEMISTRY OF DISEASE (OR CHEMOTHERAPY)

There are those who scoff that there can be little or no relationship between chemicals and disease. In fact, some scientists who receive grants and salaries from vested interests regularly publish attacks on "health foods" and label them as a "racket" because they are produced by people concerned about chemical pollution of foods with unnecessary and dangerous additives that do nothing except increase the shelf-life of mass-produced food-stuffs (and thereby the profit for the manufacturers). These hired hands of big industry scoff at any dangers from the chemicals added to foods and say their products are not devitalized but safer because they have been "enriched".

Simultaneously other hired hands of the big chemical industries are busy protesting that their sponsor's chemical drugs (mass produced and sold at great mark-ups of profit) are the answer to all man's sicknesses and that nobody should pay any attention to the producers of natural vitamins and food supplements who claim that these are more important for health than any chemical drug ever invented. These four parties — the health food producers, the chemical drug companies, the health-minded natural vitamins and food supplements producers, and the mass-producing big industries of processed foods, — all have something in common: they believe in the effectiveness of chemistry (either natural or synthetic) to influence human health.

WHAT IS DISEASE?

Consider what a chemistry textbook says on the subject of "Chemotherapy": "We find a close relationship between chemistry and disease. Disease is regarded as any condition of the living body which prevents its normal functioning. We have already noted that diabetes results from insufficient insulin and Addison's disease from lack of sufficient cortin. These are but a few of the many diseases that arise from the lack or the oversupply of some essential chemical produced by the body. In addition to these diseases there are those caused by germs and viruses. Germs produce waste products which are toxic to the body cells. The body has a method of protecting itself against the toxic effect of these substances by producing chemical substances called ANTIBODIES or ANTITOXINS." (p. 468, "ESSENTIALS OF CHEMISTRY", Garret, Haskins and Sisler, 1951, Ginn and Co., Boston). Note how this modern definition of disease is exactly in line with what naturopathy has been claiming for many generations: the basic cause of disease is TOXEMIA or poisoning, whether the poisons be produced by oversupply or undersupply of some body secretion or introduced from outside of the body.

If we will understand that the primary cause of organic disease is not germs but rather the toxemia which poisons our systems and weakens body defenses against germs, then we can understand better how to treat disease. We all live constantly in a "sea of germs"; only three per cent of all the known bacteria produce human disease reactions — the rest are either harmless or beneficial. (For instance, our digestive system is a veritable garden of bacteria, necessary for our digestive process). Man lives in a "sea of bacteria" but has been provided by God with a kind of natural immunity as long as his body is functioning according to its marvelous biochemical balance. Therefore, the best cure of disease is PREVENTION by maintaining body bio-chemical balance to resist infection. It is better to strengthen natural body defenses than to introduce powerful synthetic chemical drugs which may have serious side-effects and sometimes even create new diseases.

BIO-NUTRONICS AND DEFICIENCY DISEASES

The body was designed by God to arm and replenish its natural bio-chemical defenses through the proper use of live foods and herbs. We might call this live food (and herbal) therapy by a new name: BIO-NUTRONICS. Bio-nutronics is the science of applying live foods to preventing or correcting therapeutically the degenerative, toxic and deteriorative causes of systemic disease. Many diseases are capable of being cured through the proper use of live foods (or herbs). Just think of some of the common, degenerative diseases which took a tremendous toll of human lives until the key was found in proper nutrition. Think of the curse of SCURVY which slew countless seafaring men when they were deprived of foods containing Vitamin C —they literally wasted away for want of something as simple as could be supplied by a little fresh fruit juice daily (such as the famous limes which gave the name "limey" to the British seamen who had to daily receive their ration of lime juice). Think of beri-beri, a dread disease which was found to be caused simply by robbing the rice of its essential B vitamins through over-refined processing! Think of ricketts, a crippling deformity of bones starved by a vitamin D deficiency!

But not only are these well-known examples of "deficiency diseases" due to improper nutrition with its resultant imbalanced body chemistry, it has been discovered over and over again in recent years that many other degenerative, systemic diseases are affected by bio-chemical links: D.D. and tumors; high blood cholosterol and heart disease; unbalanced calcium metabolism and arthritis and rheumatism; low blood sugar and its relation to such varied symptoms as nervous irritability, asthma, and even insanity; the ever-mounting masses of evidence on the connection between air pollution toxins and such varied diseases as emphysema, bronchitis, lung cancer, and related diseases; the relationship between the poisonous toxins of cigarette smoking and cancers of the larynx, lungs, etc. Millions whose lives might have been saved are dead or now dying from the effects of chemical toxins that disrupt the delicate balance of blood chemistry and precipitate cellular malfunctions. But thousands have been cured or have had their health restored, preserved and rejuvenated by a change in their body chemistry through proper nutrition and avoidance of chemical toxins. Even mental disease is being cured through this new, bio-chemical approach. Dr. Linus Pauling, Nobel prize-winning chemist of the University of California, concludes that many mental disorders of the brain and nervous system may be especially affected by deficiencies in vitamins such as B1, B2, B6, B12, C, and folic acid.

It has only recently been discovered that millions of Americans may be suffering unnecessarily from hypoglycemia (low blood sugar) with such varied symptoms as asthma, obesity, arthritis, depression, anxiety, schizophrenia, delinquent and criminal behavior, convulsions, diabetes, alcoholism, etc., all because of the blood chemistry being thrown out of balance by adrenocortical glandular malfunction BROUGHT ON BY GOOD, OLD AMERICAN OVER-INDULGENCE IN REFINED SUGAR AND STARCHES! Millions have literally become "sugarholics" and wrecked their body chemistry through years of over-indulgence in carbohydrates and deficiency in proteins, natural vitamins and minerals, and fresh fruits and vegetables. I can testify from my own personal experience of having come down with a terrible case of asthma and having been offered only the usual palliatives by the medical profession — some drugs and powerful chemicals to alleviate the SYMPTOMS but no hope of a cure by getting at the CAUSES. Only after months of agonized suffering did I discover that my asthma was caused by hypoglycemia (low blood sugar), which had been brought on by years of over-indulgence in refined sugars and starches. Only by radically cutting out all the refined sugars and starches from my diet and replacing them with a high protein diet, massive vitamin and mineral therapy, and great quantities of fresh fruits and vegetables to re-alkalinize and normalize my body chemistry — only then was I cured! (The complete details of how I was cured from asthma as well as the full details on how many diseases are caused by vitamin and mineral deficiencies and glandular imbalance and how these things can be corrected by nutritional therapy, are contained in my new book on BIO-NUTRONICS).

HATRED CAN BE CURED ONLY BY CHRIST'S LOVE:

No medicine will cure hatred. This plague poisons the blood of millions, burdening their lives with affliction and often filling their bodies with disease. It fills years with unhappiness and shortens the length of life. It stains the soul and isolates the person from friends.
It causes more suffering than diseases for which people go to their doctors, but it will not respond to any medical treatment.
    He who would find the cure for hate must first of all accept full responsibility for what happens within his own soul. No man can just quit hating. He must begin loving, for it is impossible to make a vacuum in personality. Love must replace hatred.

—Milo L. Arnold

To make Infusions (Teas):

Usually about half ounce of leaves or flowers to a pint of water is used for an infusion. Pour boiling water over the herb and let stand for a short time, just as you would make common tea for the table. Sometimes a little sugar or honey makes the tea more palatable. An infusion or tea should be used while fresh.

Decoctions:

The virtues of hard materials, such as barks, roots, wood chips, seeds, etc., must be boiled for some time, just as you would make coffee. Porcelain or glass vessels should be used in preparing infusions and decoctions. Keep saucer over cup in which infusion is steeping. Keep cover over vessel in which decoction is boiling.

To Make Essence: Take about an ounce of the essential oil of the herb and dissolve in a pint of alcohol.

To Make Fomentations: Dip cloths or heavy towels in the infusion or decoction, wring out and apply locally to part you wish to cover.

To Make Ointments or Salve: An easy method to make a salve or ointment is to take about eight parts of vaseline or lard or any like substance and add two parts of the remedy you wish to use. Thus, if you were to make a sulphur salve you would use 8 oz. of vaseline and 2 oz. of sulphur; stir and mix well while hot and when cool you would have a regular sulphur salve ointment.

Very old method of making ointments: Boil ingredients in water until all properties are extracted. If a very strong ointment is desired, strain off the ingredients and add fresh ingredients to strained liquid and boil again. Add this watery decoction to sufficient olive oil and simmer until all the water has evaporated. Strain off the botanical (if it was boiled with olive oil). Add beeswax and enough rosin to solidify. Melt them together over a low flame and keep stirring until thoroughly mixed.

To Make Plasters: Bruise the leaves, root, or other part of the plant and place between two pieces of cloth, just as you would a mustard plaster, and apply to the surface you wish to cover.

To Make Poultices: Poultices are used to apply heat (moist heat), to soothe or to draw. Usually a soft substance is used, such as soap and sugar, bread and milk, mustard. etc. Some cause a counter-irritation, some draw the blood from a congested part and thus relieve pain.

To Make Syrups: After preparing the substance for a tea. boil for some time, then add 1 oz. of glycerin, and seal up in bottles or cans as you would fruit.

To Make Tincture: Take 1 oz. of the powdered herb and add 4 oz. of water and 12 oz. of alcohol. Let stand for 2 weeks. A teaspoonful of glycerin may be added. After standing for 2 weeks. pour off liquid and bottle for use. Should the herb used have a very weak medicinal power, 1 to 4 oz. of the herb may be used for the above amount of water and alcohol.

(Selected)

A most healthful and satisfying drink can be made from the fresh, raw juices of vegetables or fruits. Raw juices taken on an empty stomach will be absorbed by the blood stream and glands within 15 minutes after ingestion. A daily pint or more of rich, raw vegetable (or fruit) juices will help restore and rejuvenate an auto-intoxicated system; it would be senseless to merely add the raw juice to an already unnatural, artificial diet — instead it should REPLACE processed and preserved foods. A delicious, refreshing raw juice "cocktail" combining five or six of the above juices at a time, plus others as well (such as Beet, Pepper, Spinach), is beneficial. One popular recipe is Dr. H. E. Kirschner's therapeutic GREEN DRINK: 8 ounces of unsweetened Pineapple juice, 15 Almonds, 4 pitted Dates, 5 teaspoonfuls of Sunflower Seeds (soaked overnight in water) — liquify all of these and pour the mixture into a pitcher; next, juice four large handfuls of green leaves (such as Alfalfa, Parsley, Mint, Spinach, Beet Greens, Water-cress, Comfrey — do not use the stems) and combine with the first pitcher, stirring together. Any book on the contents of raw juices will help you to mix a healthful juice cocktail to your own taste and benefit.

Were we only to look at disease as being due to the presence of something (a germ, a virus, etc.), we would miss the vital truth that most diseases are due to the absence of something necessary in our bodies to fight off infections and parasites. More often the sick person is the victim not of what comes into his body from the outside but of what he has failed to provide inside his body. Deficiency diseases can be prevented or cured by supplying the protective food factors (vitamins, minerals, hormones, enzymes). The richest source of these protective factors is from raw foods, fresh and uncontaminated, from plants and herbs. Dr. Bircher-Benner of Switzerland wrote in 1936: "Absorption and organization of sunlight, the essence of life, takes place almost exclusively within the plants. The organs of the plant are therefore, a kind of biological accumulation of light. They are the basis of what we call food, whence animal and human bodies derive their substance and energy. Nutritional energy may thus be termed organized sunlight energy. Hence sunlight is the driving force of the cells of our body." Subsequent scientific experiments have proved that live foods contain more light radiations. Raw juices are the life blood of the fruit and vegetables, full of the vital enzymes, hormones, vitamins, minerals.

It has been well said by Dr. Robert McCarrison, "Of all the medicine created out of the earth, food is the chief." The Bible reminds us frequently that THE LIFE IS IN THE BLOOD. The juice of the plant, like the human body's blood, contains all the elements that build and nourish and protect. All foods must become liquid before our bodies can assimilate them anyway so the drinking of fresh, raw fruit and vegetable juices is the quickest and most efficient way to absorb the vital elements of plants, unchanged and unspoiled by cooking. When we eat great amounts of animal food (meats, fish, etc.) we are after all only getting the vital elements second-hand, filtered through the animal flesh. Then we must cook the animal flesh and this further cuts down the vital element. It has been well said: "No pharmacist will ever compound a pill, patent medicine or drug that can compare in curative value with the value found in uncooked, pure fruit and vegetable juices." Hippocrates, the 'father of medicine', is reported to have said: "Leave your drugs in the chemist's pot if you can heal the patient with food!" We must remember that live foods are more beneficial — it's not the food in your life but the life in your food that really counts! A six to ten day juice diet is a powerful alterative.

Some common juice combinations most helpful in treating specific diseases are the following recipes (in which carrot juice is usually about one half or two thirds of the total of each formula): Arthritis and Rheumatism— carrots, celery, beet, cucumber, parsley, watercress; Insomnia— carrot, spinach, celery, lettuce; High Blood Pressure— carrot, cucumber, parsley, celery, beet; Asthma— carrot, spinach, celery; Liver and Gall bladder disorders— carrot, beet, parsley, cucumber, dandelion, radish (about one third of total); Ulcer— comfrey, cabbage, celery, carrot; Migraine— carrot, spinach, celery, parsley.

Raw juice diets are very beneficial in most all sicknesses and should not only be used as a curative but as a preventive. But such a simple prescription goes counter to most people's habits of eating. Dr. Alexander Bryce has said: "Nothing offends patients more than to interfere with their habits of life; their desire is to break every known law of nature and when they get sick then accept complete absolution in a bottle or two of medicine — they merely want to be patched up sufficiently so they can go right back to their former habits of self-indulgence in its various forms."

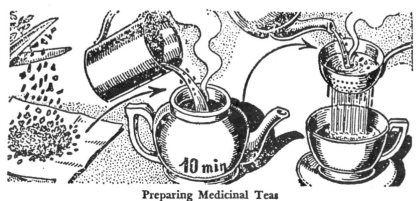

Preparing Medicinal Teas

Ecologists are warning us now that mankind is polluting his environment with tens of thousands of synthetic substances, many of which almost totally resist decay and persist on to poison man and nature— hard pesticides, metal wastes, radioactive by-products, chemical fertilizers, poisonous gases and exhaust fumes multiplying in the air, oils and detergents polluting the streams, lakes and oceans. It is the belief of this writer that modern medicine is using many questionable synthetic drugs which could be better replaced by organic herbal medicines. Organic herbal medicines are more easily assimilable and have in general less chance of leaving persistent, harmful side-effects. It is not the contention of this book that doctors can be replaced by herbs but rather that God-given herbs can greatly benefit mankind. We hope this book will serve as an introduction to whet the reader's appetite to learn more of the healthful properties of herbs both in medicine and nutrition.

If modern science were to deliberately turn its back on the healing substances waiting to be found all around us in nature, and concentrate solely on producing more artificial chemicals, the end will be sad indeed. Pesticides and air pollution have already caused an amazing rain of death to fall upon modern civilization. Since tetraethyl lead was first introduced as an automobile fuel additive in 1923, lead has contaminated most of the earth's surface. Increasing amounts of the metal are found in surface ocean waters, in crops, and in human blood, in which, in some areas, the amount may be approaching toxic levels. Excess nitrates from chemical fertilizers are contaminating the water tables in many areas. Herbicides continue to be used with wild abandon to destroy weeds and then creep into the growing crops to affect the people that eat the crops. (Emerson said that a weed is what we call a plant for which we have not yet discovered a use; it is ironic that man is poisoning weeds to produce more crops and the crops then contain more poison weakening man's whole system and then man turns to the "weeds" to find healthful herbs to combat the degenerative systemic diseases such as cancer which were aggravated and provoked by the pesticides and herbicides, chemical additives and pollutants). Even one of the Great Lakes, Lake Erie, has been overwhelmed by pollutants and DIED. Albert Schweitzer was pessimistic about man's ability to correct his scientific madness and said: "Man has lost the capacity to foresee and forestall. He will end by destroying the earth." What puny man in his scientific pride forgets is that the Bible says it will be God Who will finally have to intervene and bring civilization's mad career to a halt, in order to "DESTROY THEM WHICH DESTROY THE EARTH." (Rev. 11:18). The time cannot be much farther off at the present rate of madness.

As the Good Book, the Bible, says, the conclusion of the whole matter is that man should fear God and keep His commandments. The more man understands and uses the God-given benefits of nature, instead of polluting, destroying and trying to ignore nature and its laws, the better it will be for man. Happy the man whose medicine is his food. The secret of natural healing is symbolically referred to in the elements of the Christian ordinances or sacraments: WATER, the great cleanser and purifier (Baptism and Feet Washing); OIL, the great volatile symbol of the Holy Spirit's purity and holiness (Anointing with Oil); GRAPE JUICE, the fresh or new "wine" of Communion, unfermented, uncorrupted, typical of God-given fruits to purify man's blood and body; BREAD, typical of God-given plants or herbs that pour out of their seeds the Bread of Life for mankind in true Communion with God. Happy are those who realize that the health of the body is more than meat and drink, and true life is more than bread. Man shall not live by bread alone but by every Word that proceeds out of the Word of God. This life is only an anteroom to eternity. Happy the man who lives simply and naturally, loving God and his neighbors and hating and injuring no one. Like a tree planted beside the rivers of water, he shall bring forth fruit in his season and prosper under God's blessing, and at the end greet death not as an enemy but as a friend sent to summon him to an endless life with God in eternity.

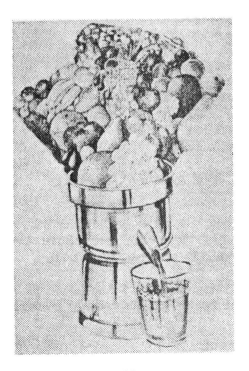

Live Fruit
and
Vegetable
Juices
Cure

APPENDIX:
Where to find Herbs, Herb Books, and Herb Doctors, and a Cross-Index of the Ailments mentioned in this book and their Herbal Remedies:

A. *Where to Find the Herbs Discussed in This Book:*

For the readers armed with unlimited time and patience and several good herbal identification books, it is an adventure to go out and collect your own herbs and then prepare them yourself. For those with less time and ambition, herbs (or homeopathic medicines based on herbs), can be purchased from:

S. Chupp's Herbs & Vitamins
27539 Londick, Dept. BKG
Burr Oak, Mich. 49030-9746

They have a large catalog of Herbs & Vitamins, Capsules & Bulk. It's free. $1.00 postage appreciated.

B. *Where to Order the Herb Books Mentioned in this Book:*

Tobe's, St. Catherine's, Ontario, Canada.

S. Chupp's Herbs & Vitamins
Dept. BKG
27539 Londick
Burr Oak, Mich. 49030

Let's Live Magazine $1.50 per issue available from S. Chupp.

"FITNESS AND HEALTH FROM HERBS", Newman Turner Publ. Ltd., Deanrow, Pasture Road, Letchworth, Herts., England ($4 per year, 12 issues).

"LET'S LIVE" Magazine, 6015 Santa Monica Blvd., Los Angeles, Cal. 90038, ($5 per year, 12 issues).

C. *Where to Find Homeopathic Physicians:*

Send to American Institute of Homeopathy, 2726 Quebec Street, N.W., Washington, D.C. 20008, and ask for their directory. Enquire in your local vicinity for naturopathic and herbalist practitioners.

D. *Index of Sicknesses and Treatments Discussed:*

For the convenience of the reader in referring back to where the various sicknesses and their herbal treatments are discussed this index is furnished. It is good to keep in mind that every more complex ailment discussed, such as rheumatism, is usually not susceptible of cure by one specific herb but that reasonable treatment must take into account avoiding the factors leading up to the disease, improvement of diet, inner cleanliness, psychological attitude, etc. What may specifically help one person's condition may need additional therapy in the case of another person. There is no cure-all except God working through nature, and nature's ways are manifold.

INDEX OF ILLNESSES DISCUSSED

Flu: 48, 54
Fractures: 61
Fungus: 36, 67

Gall bladder trouble: 59, 60, 62, 64, 77, 79
Gangrene: 48
Gas: 52, 59, 63, 65
Germs: 5, 52, 55, 59, 63
Glands: 61, 71
Gluttony: 10, 25
Goiter: 62
Gout: 40

Headaches: 51, 79
High blood-pressure: 62, 79
Hoarseness: 71
Hook-worm: ˙48, 49
Hyperactivity: 63

Iatrogenic disease: 11
Insect repellent: 51, 67
Insomnia: 27, 74, 77
Intestinal infections: 48, 51

Kidney ailments: 56, 59, 60, 61, 63, 64

Labor pains: 51
Liver trouble: 59, 63, 76, 79
Lungs: 28, 58, 61, 68, 70

Miscarriage: 51
Mouth wash: 56, 57, 77
Muscular tensions: 50

Nervous system: 55, 69, 74
Nervousness: 18, 63, 69
Neuralgia, neuritis: 61, 71, 72
Non-toxic insecticides: 67

Obesity (overweight): 32, 58, 63, 75

Parasitism: 49
Perspiration: 28, 62, 76
Phlegm: 62, 67, 71
Pimples: 52, 51
Poisons: 28, 65, 67, 69, 70, 75
Poison ivy: 67
Pregnancy problems: 50, 51
Prostrate: 64, 71
Ptomaine poisoning: 48
Pulmonary infections: 51, 56, 68, 70

Rats: 40
Respiratory system: 56, 61, 68, 71
Rheumatism: 33, 34, 35, 36, 49, 50, 55, 56, 61, 73, 77, 79, 83

Sciatica: 61, 72
Scurvy: 50
Sepsis: 51
Sins and psychosomatic sickness: 6, 7, 8, 10, 14, 16, 18, 29, 86
Sleeplessness: 27, 74, 77, 79
Spasms: 40, 50
Sore throat: 48, 54, 57, 61
Staphylococcus: 48
Stomach ache: 59, 65, 72
Stomach cramps: 59, 72
Streptococcus: 48
Sunburn: 66
Sweat glands blocked: 28, 63, 76

Tension stress: 6, 7, 8, 27, 29, 58, 62, 69
Thyroid: 62, 63
Tiredness: 69
Tooth ache: 73
Toxic wastes: 28, 34, 35, 53, 63, 73
Tuberculosis: 48, 56
Tumors: 61

Ulcers: 42, 61, 72, 79
Uric acid excess: 33, 63, 64
Urination: 56, 63, 64, 65

Viruses: 47, 48
Vitamin - mineral deficiency: 20, 25, 30, 31, 42, 50, 77
Vomiting: 65

Warts: 67, 72, 74, 77
Wasp stings: 51
Whooping cough: 56, 72
Worms: 48, 49, 65
Wounds: 42, 72, 76
Worry: 69

A FEW OUTSTANDING MEDICINAL FOODS:

Apple: valuable for its vitamin and mineral content and tendency to reduce tension; apple cider vinegar is strongly recommended for stomach, kidneys, liver.

Asparagus: a tasty, powerful diuretic.

Avocado: delicious fruit tending to reduce cholesterol level in the blood.

Cabbage: the juice contains a high vitamin and mineral content — a good cleanser.

Carrots: high in vitamins, especially good as a purifying juice diet.

Celery: a sedative and calmative, especially in the juice.

Cherry: relieves arthritic and rheumatic conditions, especially the juice.

Citrus fruits: generally beneficial for high Vitamin C content in all rheumatic conditions, kidneys, etc. Diaphoretic when taken hot.

Cucumbers: a diuretic food, also refrigerant.

Figs: a good food and an excellent laxative and purifier.

Grapes: a blood purifier (especially in the exclusive grape diet or Grape Cure).

Garlic and Onion: two marvellous vegetable anti-biotics; raw onion will cure sores on the tongue and in the mouth.

Lettuce: soporific or sleep-inducing action.

Parsley: cleanser and sedative, to be taken only in small quantities when juiced.

Papaya: a good digestant, rich in enzymes, also a good poultice for burns, warts, freckles, pimples, etc.

Quince: simmer the seed in water to produce a good mouth wash or burn dressing.

Radish: marvelous when combined with other vegetables in juice, a purifier, especially for gall bladder.

Rhubarb: a safe and effective laxative.

Watercress: good for eczema, night blindness, soft teeth and weak bones.

Watermelon: strong in the bioflavonoids and a good diuretic.

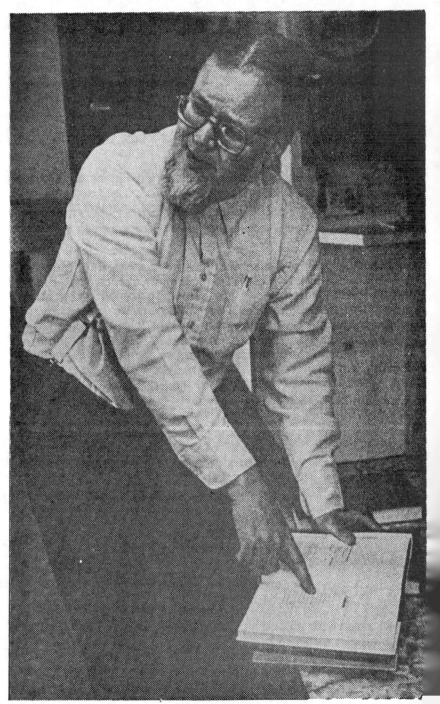

The Author

AMISH FOLK REMEDIES
by William McGrath

A best seller, explaining Amish Traditions, their proven Herbal Formulas used for generations to stay healthy, happy and stay youthful. Most formulas are available in Herb Gardens or Health Stores. Makes a nice Gift! PG Formula's are given for a fast easy delivery used by the Amish women.

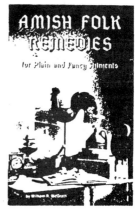

AMERICAN INDIAN FOLK REMEDIES

by William McGrath - Covers over 140 herbs used by the Indians including Pau d'Arco Tea used by many for the incurables! Tells of teas used to overcome impotence, prostate, weight problems, arthritis and much more!

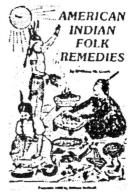

GOD GIVEN HERBS
by William McGrath

New printing - 1986 - by request First distributor ordered 500 books! Ailments from Arthritis, cancer to whooping cough. Remedies given. This Book tells on pages 33 & 34 how he was cured from crippleling rheumatoid arthritis, using simple home remedies!

GOD-GIVEN HERBS
FOR THE HEALING
OF MANKIND

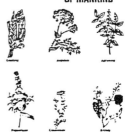

S. Chupp's Books
27539 Londick
Burr Oak, Mich. 49030

Notes

Notes

Notes